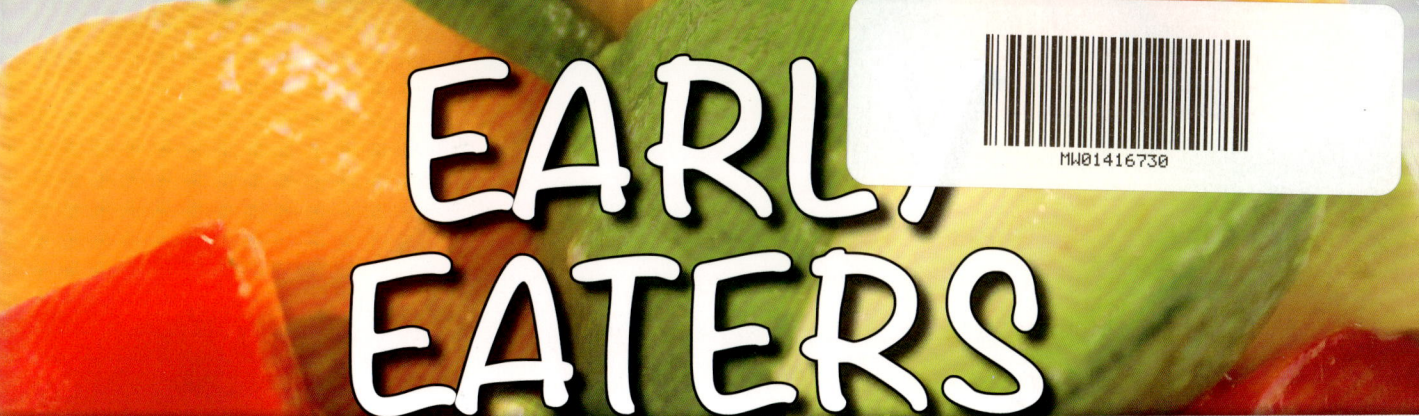

EARLY EATERS

survival tips and simple recipes for toddlers and preschoolers

CONTENTS

Get ready to raise a healthy eater 2

Mealtime does not have to be stressful 4

MyPlate.. 8

Extra jars or pouches of baby food 10

Introducing new foods to toddlers – the 10x rule................. 11

Turning picky eaters into healthy eaters.......................... 12

Making the most of your child's day 14

The basics of taste – balancing "the buds" 18

Junior chef kitchen activities 20

Cooking terms 22

Let's get cooking 24

Kitchen safety... 25

Recipes... 26

Get ready to raise a healthy eater

Congratulations, you have just started your journey to raising a healthy eater! Unlocking the likes and dislikes of early eaters (toddlers and preschoolers) during this period of extreme growth can be exhausting. We know you are busy. We want to give you the best tips and tricks to help save time and energy.

During early childhood (ages 1-4 years old), growth rates start to slow down compared to when your child was an infant. This means their appetite will decrease. The amount and types of foods eaten at meals and snacks may change by the hour or day.

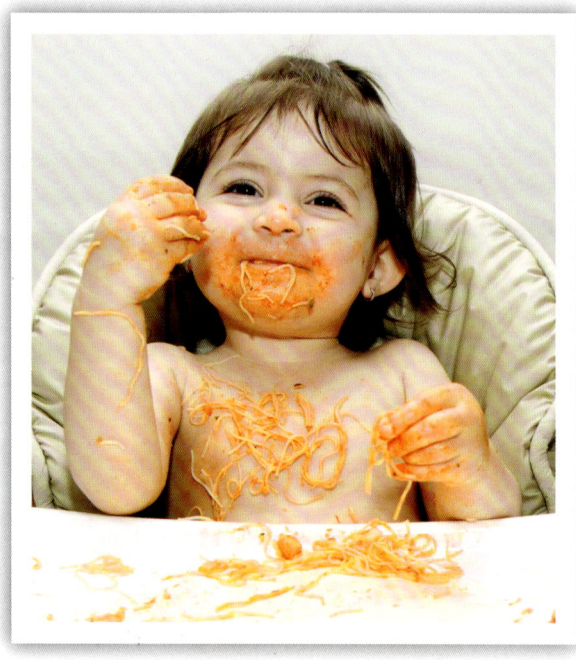

Be ready for the mess

Place a towel or old shower curtain on the floor to make cleanup easier. Have paper towels or a sponge handy. Encourage your child to help you clean up a spill. A spill is not a disaster, but rather an opportunity to help them learn.

Toddlers, children 1-2 years old, are known for their independence and sometimes by their struggles over food. Particularly, their refusal to eat some foods. They are very busy building fine motor skills. They are learning to use fingers to pick up small food pieces, pushing food onto a spoon, and drinking from a cup. Eating is almost always a messy time.

- As your toddler's eating skills develop, they can move from eating soft pieces of food to eating foods with more texture.

- Toddlers may not try new foods. They need to look, touch and smell new foods before tasting them. Even then, they still may not eat the new food the next time it is served.

- Toddlers are unpredictable. They may like certain foods one day and dislike them the next day. They may eat a lot one day and very little the next day. This may change from meal to meal too.

As children grow from toddlers to preschoolers, they begin to have a good handle on self-feeding. They may still choose to eat with their hands over using a fork or spoon. They are becoming more interested in trying new foods and start to enjoy the social part of family meals.

- Preschoolers are more curious about food than they were as toddlers. They still may be unwilling to try new foods.

- Preschoolers can serve themselves. They may be more likely to try food that they have put on their plate.

- Your child may have a very limited list of foods they are willing to eat. This is normal too!

Mealtime does not have to be stressful

There is no doubt that mealtimes with a young child can test your patience. It can also be frustrating if your child refuses to eat the healthy meal you have cooked. When this happens, the best approach is to stay calm and understand they are simply learning about food and how to act at the table. Try these simple tips to make mealtime a great experience.

BE A POSITIVE ROLE MODEL

Children learn by watching you, they look up to you and want to be just like you. One of the best ways to raise a healthy eater is to be one yourself. Here are some ideas to help you become a role model of healthy eating:

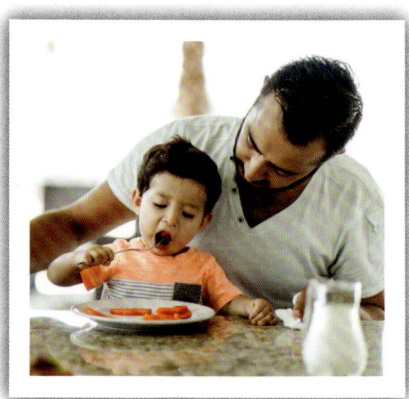

The best way to raise a healthy eater is to be one yourself.

- Keep a rainbow of fruits and vegetables on hand and ready to eat, instead of salty or sugary snacks.

- Cook foods in healthier ways, such as baking, grilling, roasting and steaming. Limit deep-frying.

- Drink water, instead of soda or sugary drinks.

- Buy only some processed foods. Read labels to choose products that have common ingredients found in your kitchen, not in a chemistry lab.

- Make fast food and junk food "once-in-a-while" foods. These foods are high in fat, salt, and calories.

FAMILY MEALS SHOULD INCLUDE A VARIETY OF HEALTHY FOOD CHOICES

Parenting has many jobs, but a custom order cook is not one of them. Save time, money and stress by making one healthy meal for the family. It can be upsetting if your child does not eat much of the meal. Do not give in to them asking for special foods. Your child will learn the right way to behave by watching the rest of the family eat the meal.

For main meals, serve new foods along with 1-2 foods that you know your child will eat. Offering 1-2 foods you know your child likes gives you clues to their hunger. If they eat the foods that they like, you know they are hungry and may be more willing to try the new foods too.

Children often do better with simple meals. For example, if you are making pasta with tomato sauce, try serving the sauce on the side instead of mixed with the pasta. This way your child can choose to try the sauce or not. If you are serving a dish with many ingredients, try separating the ingredients on the plate so they can try foods based on color, shape, and type. The key to healthy meals is variety which builds strong and healthy bodies. Throughout the day, include foods from all five food groups (see page 8) in meals and snacks.

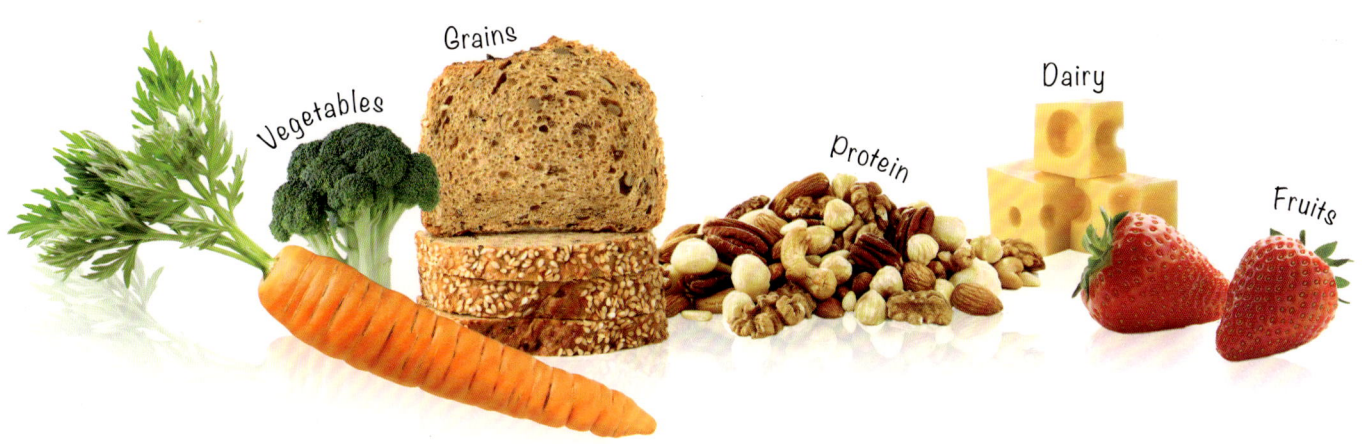

mealtime does not have to be stressful

LET YOUR CHILD DECIDE WHAT AND HOW MUCH TO EAT

During toddler and preschooler years, as your child's growth rate slows down, the types and amounts of foods eaten at meals and snacks may seem completely random. Your child was born with the skill to control the type and amount of food to eat. They know this based on signals from their own body. However, these signals can easily be stopped by emotions or demands from an adult.

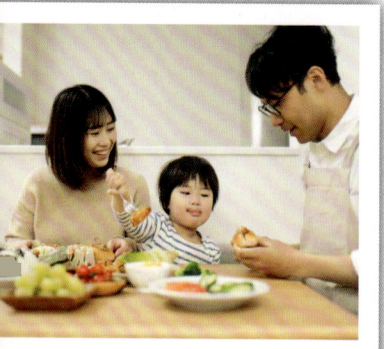

Your child should learn to listen to their body's signals. These signals will alert them when they are full. Forcing your child to finish all their food teaches them to overeat. The habit of overeating affects their ability to stop eating when they are full. Encourage your child to try the foods on the plate instead of finishing everything. If you worry about wasting uneaten food, encourage your child to take small servings and allow them to have seconds or thirds.

Encourage your child to try the foods on the plate instead of finishing everything.

MEALTIME IS FAMILY TIME

Think of this time as a change from feeding your child to eating with your child. Even if your family is a small number of people, it is important to enjoy each other by sharing meals together. Make mealtime warm and relaxing. Teach your child mealtime manners and what behaviors are best at the table. When your child feels good and knows how to act around food, sooner or later they will learn to eat almost everything you eat.

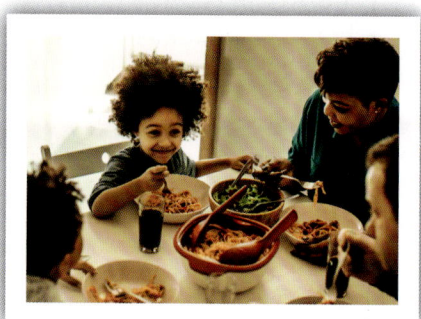

Serve meals family style.

To make family mealtime enjoyable try to:
- Eat at a table, not in front of the TV.
- Put away phones, tablets, and papers.
- Play slow, quiet music during meals.
- Serve meals family style with each person making their plate from the food choices offered.
- Talk about fun and happy topics. Ask questions about the favorite parts of your child's day.

mealtime does not have to be stressful

MAKE FOOD FUN

Nothing makes a toddler or preschooler happier than helping an adult. So why not teach your child to be a smart shopper or junior chef? Children who help pick out and prepare foods are more willing to try new foods.

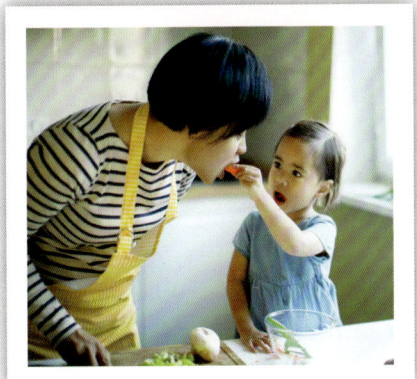

When you are at the grocery store, have your child pick out colorful fruits and vegetables. Teach them how to look for good-looking produce. Ask them to help you find a food, like broccoli or sweet potatoes. Asking questions, like "Do you want to eat carrots or cauliflower for dinner?" allows them to be included in decisions at the store. This makes it more likely they will try these foods at the table.

Have your child be a kitchen helper. There are plenty of activities that your child can do to help in the kitchen (see page 20). Having a hand in the preparation can build excitement for the meal.

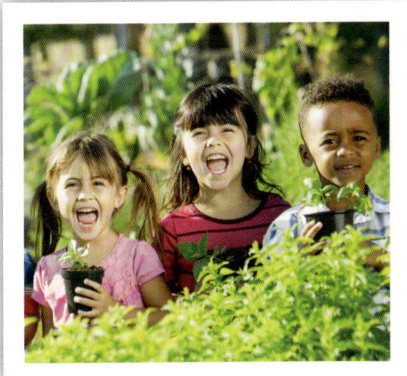

Try growing food. You do not need a big garden to teach a child where food comes from. A simple recycled container in the window can do the trick. A little dirt, a few plant seeds, water, and sunshine are all you need to watch the magic of nature happen.

At mealtime, make a game of saying the names of the colors and the foods, like "Who can name the red food on the plate?". Colorful eating is an easy idea to teach small children. The game will go a long way toward developing healthy, positive eating habits.

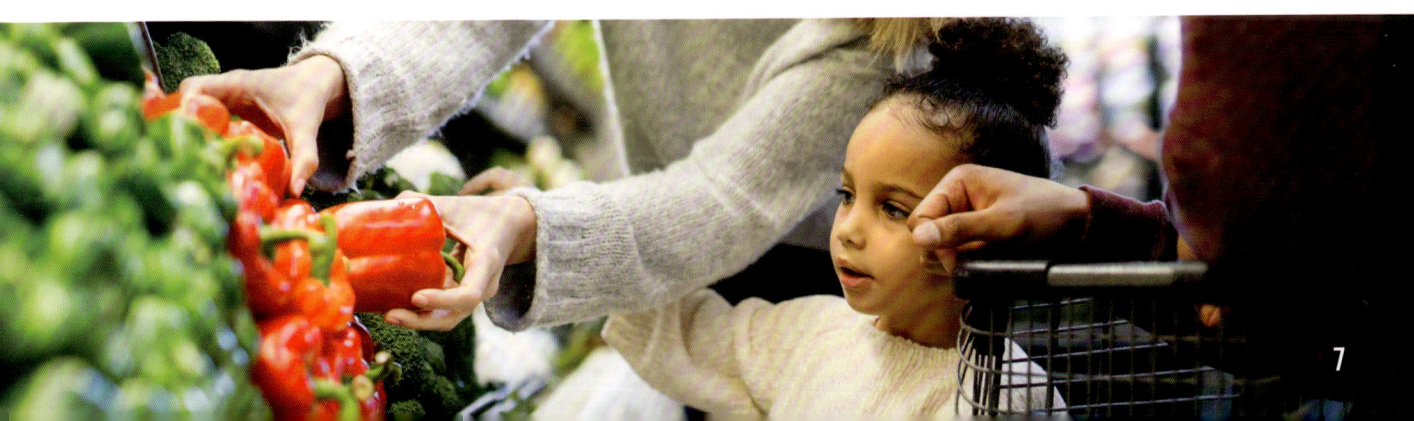

MyPlate

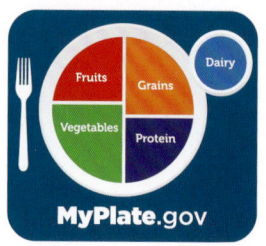

There are five food groups that make up the building blocks for a healthy diet. When grocery shopping and making meals, the MyPlate picture is an easy way to remember these foods groups. It is not necessary to have every food group represented at each meal. Try to eat and serve foods from all five of the food groups each day.

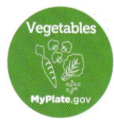

VEGETABLE GROUP
VARY YOUR VEGGIES

 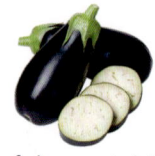 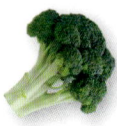

Brighten your child's plate with a variety of colorful vegetables at meals and snacks. Vegetables may be fresh, frozen, canned, or dried, and may be whole, cut-up, or pureed. If you choose canned vegetables, be sure that they are labeled as "reduced sodium" or "no-salt-added." Some raw vegetables can be hard, making them choking hazards for small children. Try serving these ones, such as carrots, boiled, baked or steamed.

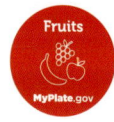

FRUIT GROUP
FOCUS ON WHOLE FRUITS

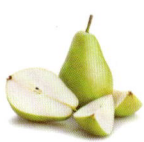 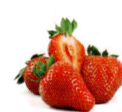 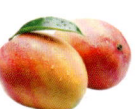

Include a rainbow of fruits in your child's meals or snacks. Fruits can be fresh, frozen, canned, or dried, and may be whole, cut-up, or pureed. If you choose canned fruits, be sure that they are packed in water or 100% juice instead of syrup because syrup adds sugar and calories. Some fruits, such as grapes, are a choking hazard for small children.

Toddlers who drink fruit juice are more likely to have tooth decay and less likely to drink water as they grow older. If you want to offer your child fruit juice, choose 100% fruit juice. Check the ingredient label to be sure. Limit daily servings to ½ cup (4 ounces) for children 1-3 years old and ½ - ¾ cup (4 to 6 ounces) for children 4-6 years old.

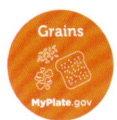

GRAIN GROUP
MAKE HALF YOUR GRAINS WHOLE

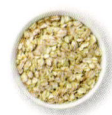 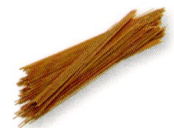 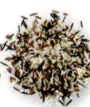

Eating grains, such as whole-grain bread, cereals, rice, and pasta, provides health benefits and nutrients, including fiber. Read ingredient labels and choose foods that name one of the following whole-grain ingredients first:

brown rice	oatmeal	barley	whole-grain triticale	whole wheat
buckwheat	quinoa	whole-grain corn	whole oats	wild rice
bulgur	rolled oats	whole-grain sorghum	whole rye	
millet	whole-grain			

Note: Foods labeled with the words "multi-grain," "stone-ground," "100% wheat," "cracked wheat," "seven-grain," or "bran" may not be whole-grain products. With whole grain products, you get the complete benefit of the wheat plant, rather than pieces or parts which may not provide you with the full health benefits.

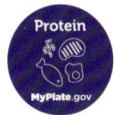

PROTEIN GROUP
VARY YOUR PROTEIN ROUTINE

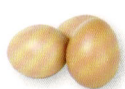 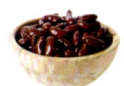 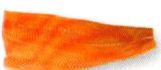

Introduce your child to a variety of protein foods — including seafood, meat, poultry, eggs, beans and peas, soy products, nuts and seeds. Select lean meat and poultry. Choose fish that is lower in mercury such as Salmon, Flounder, Tilapia, Trout, Pollack, and Catfish. Limit highly processed poultry, fish, or meat (like hotdogs, chicken nuggets, and fish sticks). Nuts and seeds, other than finely ground, can be a choking hazard for a young child.

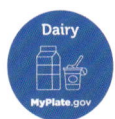

DAIRY GROUP
MOVE TO LOW-FAT OR FAT-FREE MILK OR YOGURT

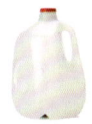  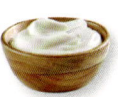

Dairy provides health benefits like building strong bones and teeth. Good dairy choices include milk, yogurt, cheese, and vitamin-fortified soymilk. Whole milk is recommended for 1-year-old toddlers. Switch to fat-free (skim) or low-fat dairy choices when your child turns 2. Children over 2 should drink unflavored milk most often because flavored milk is high in added sugar.

Extra jars or pouches of baby food

Has your baby become a toddler overnight and left you with unopened jars of baby food? Here are a few ideas the help use up this food instead of letting it go to waste.

FRUIT BABY FOODS
such as apple, peaches, and pears

1. Sweeten plain yogurt with fruit baby food.
2. Add fruit baby food to smoothies.
3. Mix fruit purees into unsweetened applesauce.
4. Spread fruit baby food on toast.
5. Use fruit baby food as a dip with baby-safe crackers.

VEGETABLE BABY FOODS
such as butternut squash, peas, and carrots

1. Add vegetable baby food to tomato sauce. Mix it with pasta or use it to make pizzas.
2. Use vegetable baby food like sauce. Spoon them over brown rice or pieces of chopped meat.
3. Add sweet potato or butternut squash baby food to pancake batter.
4. Mix vegetable baby food into mashed potatoes or macaroni and cheese.
5. Add vegetable baby food to meatloaf or meatballs.

MEAT BABY FOODS
such as chicken, turkey or beef

1. Add meat purees into vegetable soup recipes.
2. Combine meat baby food and baby cereal to make mini-meatballs or slider hamburgers.
3. Use baby food meat purees to make savory muffins with meat, veggies, and cheese.

DRY BABY CEREAL

1. Use baby cereal in place of bread crumbs in any recipe.
2. Add baby cereal to yogurt or smoothies for a thicker texture.
3. Use baby cereal to thicken a sauce or gravy.

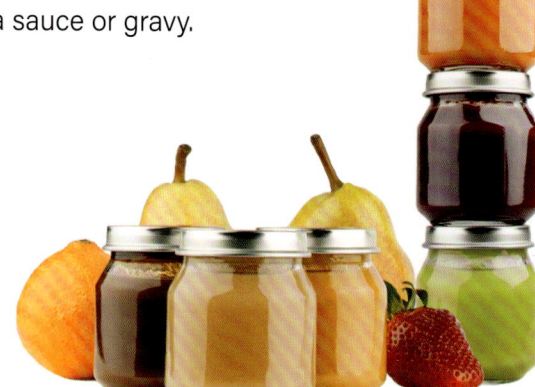

Introducing new foods to toddlers – the 10x rule

Is your toddler unwilling to try new foods? Here's why. The American Academy of Pediatrics performed a study with toddlers and found that most toddlers need to see a new food on their plate at least 10 times before they are willing to try it. Try these tips for introducing new foods more successfully:

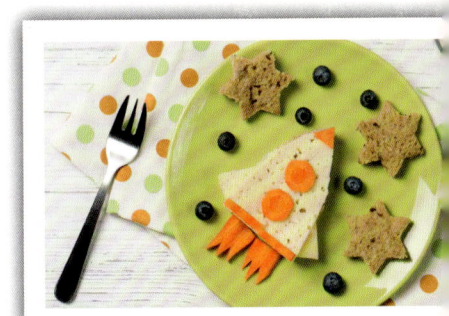

1. **Offer new foods first.** Your child is most hungry at the start of a meal. They will often eat without thinking about what they are eating.

2. **Pair a new food with familiar food.** Serve something that you know your child likes along with new food.

3. **Make food creative.** Toddlers are often open to trying new foods arranged in eye-catching and creative ways. Use cookie cutters to cut foods into shapes or arrange foods by colors. Kids this age also enjoy any food involving a dip.

4. **Talk about the new food.** Introduce a food and describe the flavor and texture. Compare it to a food they already like.

5. **It is fun to try it.** Be a good role model and show your child how you enjoy trying a new food.

6. **Try serving new food at different times of the day.** Does your child eat the most at breakfast? Could this new food be a snack? Try offering the new food at other times of the day to encourage trying.

It is the parent's responsibility to provide healthy food, and the child's decision to eat it.

Turning picky eaters into healthy eaters

Picky eating is common for most early eaters. It is a normal part of growing up. If your child is growing as the doctor suggests, they are most likely eating enough to be healthy. If you have concerns about your child's growth or eating behavior, ask for advice from their healthcare provider. Otherwise join the group of many parents and caregivers, who are working through the challenges of living with a picky eater.

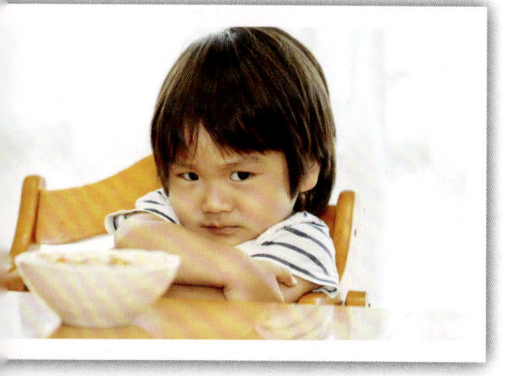

"Sam will not eat anything green"

"Julia will not try any new foods."

"Chantelle has gone days on macaroni and cheese."

"Miguel used to eat carrots every day, and he just stopped eating them."

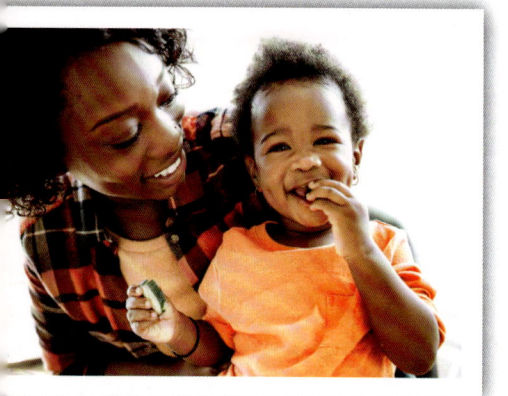

Do you any of these comments remind you of your little one?
YOU ARE NOT ALONE.

12 turning picky eaters into healthy eaters

The best reaction is no reaction. Make picky eating no big deal. It will likely go away before school age. This will be challenging. It is hard not to give in to your early eater's objections. Do not fall into the trap of offering bland, unhealthy foods to replace flavorful, healthy foods. Here is more advice:

Begin early: In the first 2 years of your child's life, set them up for healthy growth and development by teaching healthy habits right away.

Offer choices: Let your child make some food choices like, "Do you want broccoli or carrots for dinner?" Simple choices make your child feel in control. It is also easy to forget about healthy foods you do not like but remember to let your child try everything. Even if you are not a tomato fan, your child could love cherry tomatoes!

Start small: Be realistic about setting goals. It is not realistic to ask your child to eat a whole serving of a food that they claim not to like. Instead, start with a small goal — like one bite of the new food — and work your way up from there. Try offering just that small bite of food on the plate, so the child does not feel overwhelmed by eating a large amount.

Mix it up: How can the food be prepared? Raw or cooked; hot, cold, or frozen; plain or with a dipping sauce; whole or cut up? Asking your child how they would like their food prepared provides them with control to make decisions.

Try pairing flavors: Early eaters tend to prefer sweet and salty flavors and dislike sour and bitter flavors. Putting these flavors together will please an early eater's taste buds. For example, serve broccoli (bitter) with melted cheese (salty).

Celebrate the wins: Congratulate your child, even if they have just had a nibble. For a picky eater, a little nibble is a big deal.

Time is your friend: Do not punish or bribe your child if they do not eat new foods right away. Some children just need a little more time to try new foods.

Making the most of your child's day

BREAKFAST

Eating a good breakfast sets your child up for the day. Studies show that children who eat this meal have a lower risk of becoming overweight and they perform better at school. Eating breakfast will help them learn more and behave better. Here are a few tips for breakfast success:

- A healthy breakfast includes protein, whole grains, fruits or vegetables, and dairy.
- Keep TV and screens turned off during the meal.
- Prepare breakfast foods in advance and freeze them in single servings. They can quickly defrost in the microwave or the toaster oven.
- Have "on the go" breakfast items, like small boxes of whole-grain cereals, fresh fruits, yogurt in the tube and granola bars on hand. You can bring them to-go if you are running late.

LUNCH

The secret to a great lunch is keeping it simple and offering choices. This approach is easy for you to make and your child will enjoy the choices. Many lunch foods can be prepared in advance in large quantities. Each morning fill small containers with 3-4 food choices. Easy lunch choices include:

- Applesauce (look for no sugar added on the label)
- Celery sticks filled with cream cheese or peanut butter sprinkled with raisins
- Cheese cubes or cut string cheese logs
- Dried fruit
- Fresh fruit pieces or a piece of whole fruit
- Hard-boiled egg (peeled)
- Hummus with carrots and mini pita bread
- Lunch meat rolled up
- Peanut butter with apple slices
- Sugar snap peas, carrots, or cucumber slices with ranch dressing
- Whole-grain crackers or pretzels
- Yogurt or a smoothie

SAFE FOOD IN A SAFE SETTING

Your child's meals and snacks should always be eaten while they are sitting and with an adult watching. Take precautions against choking. Offer foods that are bite-sized and soft enough to chew easily. Recipes made at home or store-bought foods may need to be mashed or cut into small pieces. Be cautious of foods your child can choke on: raw hard vegetables, whole grapes, peanut butter, chips, nuts, popcorn, dried fruits, hot dogs, chunks of meat, and hard candy. Some safety suggestions include: steam hard vegetables, cut grapes in half and spread peanut butter thinly.

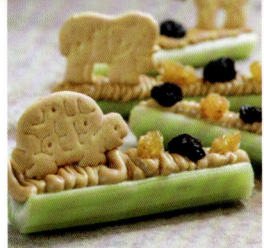

SNACK SMART

Children get hungry between meals; their tummies are a lot smaller than ours. Along with having 3 meals a day at set times, plan to offer sit-down snacks every 2 to 3 hours between mealtimes. Snacks give the body a boost of energy between meals.

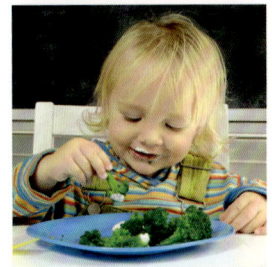

Do not confuse snacks with junk foods; they are not the same things. Instead of stocking your kitchen with chips and cookies, offer your child one of these items:

- Fresh fruit with yogurt dip
- Cut up veggies with ranch dressing
- Whole-grain crackers
- Rice cakes with a cheese slice
- Dried fruits, nuts, seeds, or trail mix
- Cookies made from real fruit or fruit juice
- Smoothies made from fresh fruit, yogurt, and sorbet
- Baked snack chips
- Hummus and pita bread
- Guacamole with corn chips or raw veggies

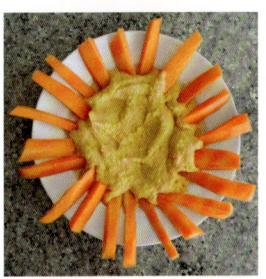

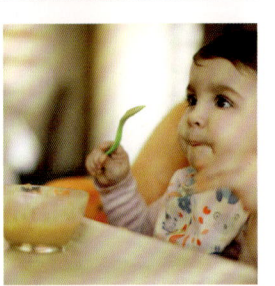

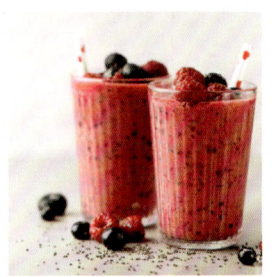

DINNER

Homemade meals are healthier and cost less than processed or restaurant meals. Making dinner can seem to be a huge chore at busy times, though. Here are a few tips to ease the stress of getting dinner on the table:

- Plan menus and make a shopping list. These two steps take a few minutes but will save time in the long run.
- Set aside time in your day off to cook foods and freeze them to eat later in the week.
- Connect with a friend to cook, doubling recipes, and splitting the dishes in half for both families to enjoy.
- Serve simple side dishes with "no-cook" items like apples, pears, avocados or tomatoes. Just wash, slice, and serve.
- Team up with a friend or neighbor to have a family dinner at their house one night and at your house on a different night.
- Make extra for leftovers. Leftovers make tasty lunches.
- When you cook up a family favorite, double the recipe and freeze a portion for a dinner next week.

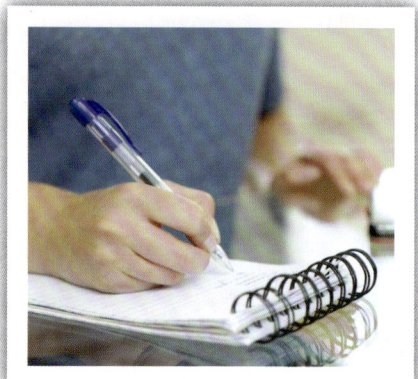 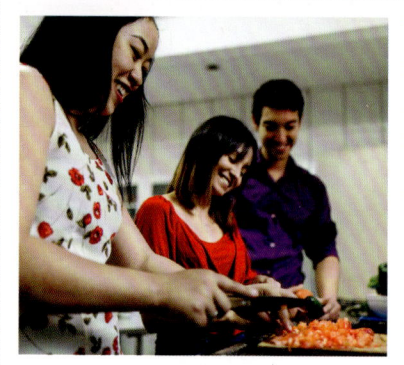 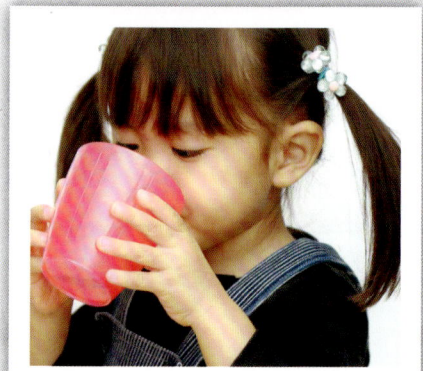

DRINK CHOICES

Water and milk are the best drink choices, and small amounts of 100% fruit or vegetable juice are fine too. Offer your child milk and juice from an open cup, not a sippy cup.

Water: When your child tells you they are thirsty, offer water to quench their thirst. Water is important to keep your child's body healthy in many ways. Plus, unlike many other drinks, water will not provide liquid calories, making it less likely that your child will feel full and not be hungry at mealtimes. This can be especially important if you have a picky eater.

Milk: Milk provides nutrients that growing children need. When your child turns 2 years old, switch to 1% (low-fat) or skim (fat-free) milk. Milk is filling. Offer your child a small cup of milk to make sure they have room for other important foods. Choose plain milk over flavored milk, like chocolate or strawberry milk. They have added sugar and calories.

Juice: Even though 100% fruit juice provides some vitamins, too much juice can lead to weight gain, diarrhea, and tooth decay. Your child should be offered whole fruits over juice whenever possible.

Your child does not need soda or sweetened drinks, like sports drinks, sweet teas and juice drinks. These drinks contain a lot of added sugar. They can add to weight gain and cavities in kids. They can also fill a child up, leaving no room for healthy foods.

WHAT ABOUT DESSERT?

Many parents struggle with what to do about sweets. Consider these options:

- Serve a small treat (a cookie or mini muffin) with your child's dinner. Allow them to eat it first if they choose. Over time, your child will learn that sweets are part of the meal but not the only part.

- Serve a small treat at the end of the meal regardless of how much your child has eaten. This removes dessert from being a special reward.

- Eliminate sweets altogether and do not start the habit of expecting a sweet to end the meal.

The basics of taste – balancing "the buds"

Taste buds are our balancing boards of flavor. The five basic tastes are: salty, sour, bitter, sweet and the newcomer called umami. These tastes work together to create flavors that are yummy, yucky, and everything in between.

SALTY

Salty foods enhance flavor and increase thirst and appetite.

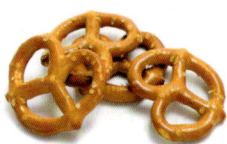

EXAMPLES

table salt, pretzels, crackers, bacon, and capers.

SOUR

Sour foods are refreshing and quench thirst. Sour foods tend to "brighten up" the taste of a dish.

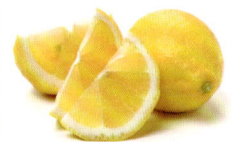

EXAMPLES

tomatoes, lemons, limes, pickles, vinegar, mustard, green apples, and yogurt.

BITTER

Bitter foods increase hunger. Bitterness is the most sensitive of the tastes and is thought by many to be unpleasant or sharp.

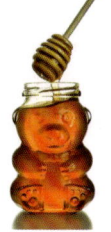

EXAMPLES

leafy greens (i.e. kale, collard, chard, etc.), brussels sprouts, dark chocolate, green peppers, and olives.

SWEET

Sweet foods satisfy and make you feel full. Sweet foods find their best balance with bitter or sour foods.

EXAMPLES

sugar, honey, maple syrup, grapes, berries, onions, carrots, corn, and sweet potatoes.

UMAMI

(pronounced oo-MA-mee) Umami's taste is hard to describe, but it means earthy, meaty, or satisfying.

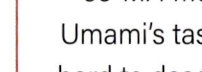

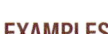

EXAMPLES

soy sauce, parmesan cheese, tomato paste, asparagus, mushrooms, nuts, and beef broth.

ENCOURAGE YOUR CHILD TO APPRECIATE THEIR TASTE BUDS

Healthy eating is all about balance and variety when it comes to helping introduce your little one to new tastes. Here are a few tips that can help expand or improve the balance in your child's taste buds.

Kitchen fun: Allow your child to experience and identify the five unique tastes that make up their taste buds. Taste small amounts of different ingredients to guess which taste group they belong to.

Stay balanced: Good taste is a balancing act. Include a variety of tastes in your meals and encourage your child to try all kinds of foods. Experiencing the same tastes all the time is not a path to healthy, adventurous eating.

Talk about it: When you hear "that is yummy!" or "yuck – that is terrible!" – ask which flavor is best or bothering. The more you understand your child's taste preferences, the easier it may be to guide and expand their food choices.

Sweet tendency: Both breast milk and formula are sweet, so it is only natural that sweet is the first taste we develop. This means that when your child begins eating solid food they may prefer sweet-tasting food. Be sure to introduce your child to other tastes early to keep a preference for sweet from overpowering their taste buds.

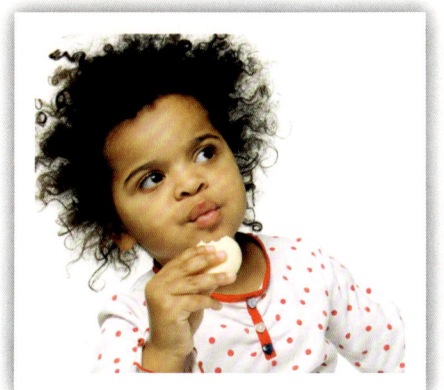
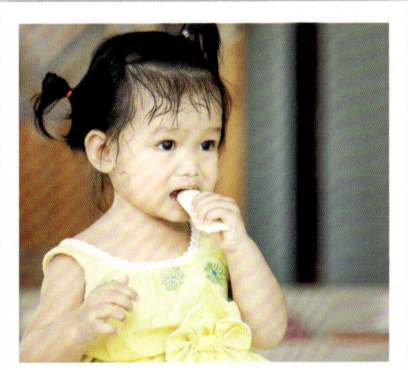
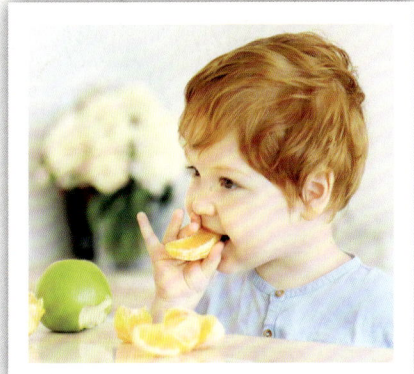

the basics of taste – balancing "the buds"

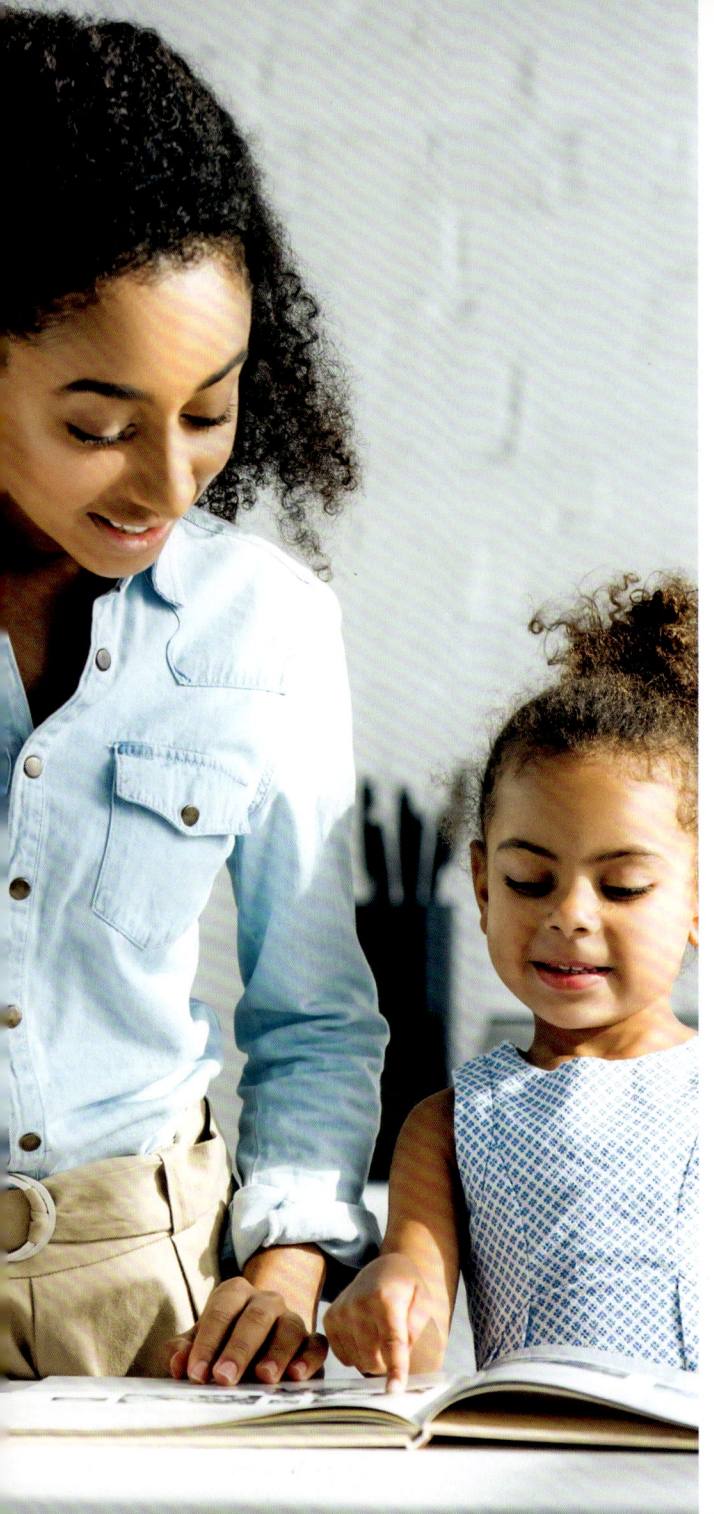

Junior chef kitchen activities

AT 2 YEARS

- Wipe tables
- Carry utensils to a table or countertop
- Place things in the trash
- Help you read a cookbook by turning the pages
- Rinse vegetables or fruits

AT 3 YEARS
All that a 2-year-old can do, plus:

- Add ingredients to a mixing bowl
- Talk about cooking
- Scoop or mash potatoes
- Squeeze citrus fruits
- Knead and shape dough
- Name and count foods
- Help put ingredients on a pizza
- Prepare fruits and vegetables without a knife (snapping beans, husking corn, tearing lettuce)

AT 4 YEARS
All that a 3-year-old can do, plus:

- Set the table
- Peel hard-cooked eggs
- Peel fruits by hand, such as oranges and bananas
- Crack eggs
- Pour liquid ingredients into a bowl of dry ingredients
- Help measure dry ingredients
- Help make sandwiches and tossed salads

AT 5 YEARS
All that a 4-year-old can do, plus:

- Use a scrub brush to clean hard fruits and vegetables
- Use measuring cups and spoons for dry and liquid ingredients
- Stir ingredients in a bowl
- Use a dull knife to spread
- Clear the table after eating

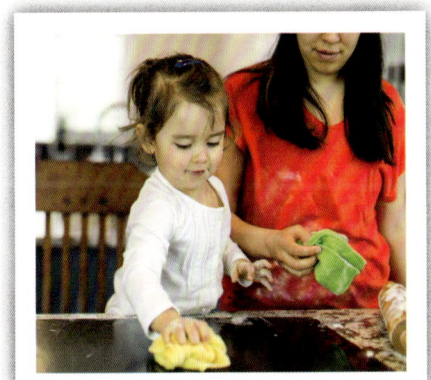
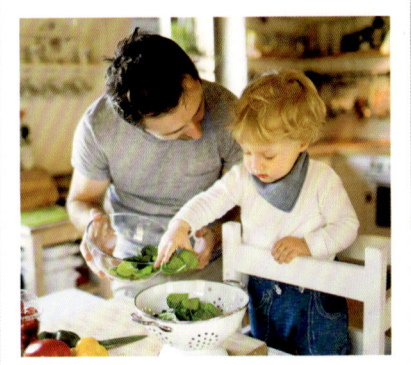
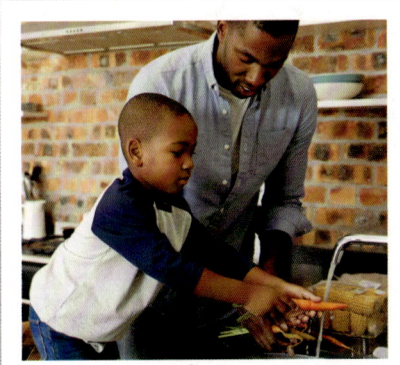

Cooking terms

The cooking directions in a recipe describe the steps for preparing the dish. The same cooking terms appear in most recipes. Here are the most common cooking terms and what they mean.

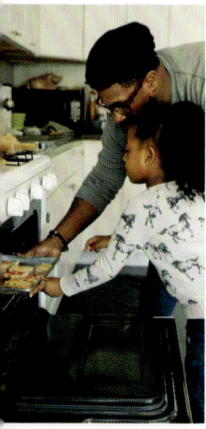

OVEN COOKING:

Bake: To cook with dry heat in an oven.

Broil: To cook directly under heat (top browning).

Grease: To coat a pan with grease, butter or cooking spray so food does not stick to it when it is placed in the pan.

Preheat: To turn on the oven and give it time to get to hot enough. This is the first step in recipes for baked foods. The oven must be hot enough for the food to cook in the time allowed. It usually takes about 10-15 minutes to preheat the oven. Turn your oven on before you get out your ingredients.

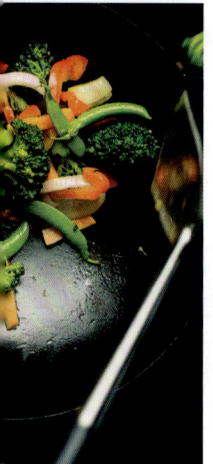

STOVETOP COOKING:

Boil: To heat a liquid on the top of the stove over high heat until it bubbles. Once a food begins to boil, you can adjust the heat to prevent the food from boiling over the top of the pot.

Brown: To cook on top of the stove quickly. Turn the burner to medium-high or high heat, place the food in the pan and turn the food so that all sides turn brown.

Sauté or Fry: (also called pan-fry) To cook with a small amount of oil or butter on top of the stove.

Simmer: To cook food on the stovetop over very low heat with the food moving but not bubbling.

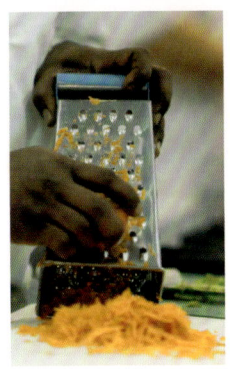

CUTTING:

Chop: To cut food into smaller pieces, usually with a large knife and cutting board.

Dice: To cut food into tiny cubes — less than 1/2 inch in size.

Grate or Shred: To shave off very small pieces using a grater.

Mince: To cut food into very small pieces.

Peel: To strip off the skin of a fruit or vegetable using a knife or vegetable peeler.

Slice: To cut food into thin pieces.

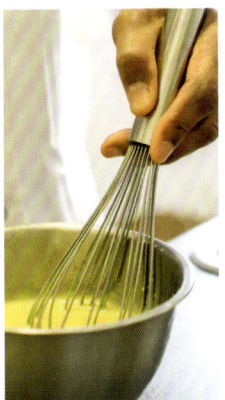

MIXING:

Beat: To stir very fast in a circular motion to create a smooth mixture. Some recipes may recommend using an electric mixer to beat the ingredients.

Combine: To mix all ingredients together.

Puree: To make food smooth and creamy, usually in a blender or food processor.

Mash: To crush food into a smooth texture.

Mix: To stir, usually with a spoon, to combine ingredients.

Whisk: To mix ingredients with a light, rapid movement, usually with a whisk.

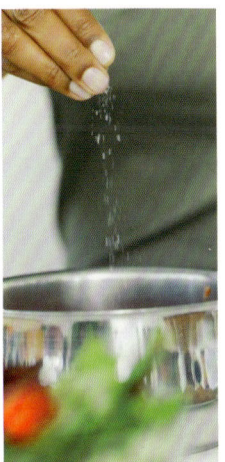

OTHER COMMON RECIPE WORDS:

Chill: To make food cold, usually by placing it in the refrigerator.

Cool: To drop the temperature of food by letting it stand at room temperature.

Cover: To put something over the top such as a pan lid, a piece of foil, or plastic wrap.

Dash or Pinch: A very small amount; less than 1/8 teaspoon.

Drain: To pour off liquid from food, often by using a colander or strainer.

Tbsp: Short for tablespoon.

tsp: Short for teaspoon.

Let's get cooking

Cooking can be fun! If you haven't spent much time in the kitchen, or even if you have and you need new ideas, these tips will help you become a cooking success.

STEPS TO TACKLE A RECIPE

Recipes are written in two parts. There is a list of ingredients and then a set of directions. Follow these easy steps:

1. Read the recipe all the way through before you start.
2. Check your supplies to make sure you have all the ingredients.
3. See that you have the right equipment for the recipe.
4. When you are ready to get started, get out all the ingredients and the equipment.
5. Follow the recipe instructions. Measure ingredients and follow cooking times.

The recipes in this book are designed with the whole family in mind and are especially kid-friendly. They are healthy and full of great flavor.

Serving sizes: This serving information is a guide to support you in making meals. There will be times when your child will not eat a whole serving and there may be times when they ask for more. The serving sizes listed in each recipe include both adult, preschooler (half of an adult serving) and toddler (half of a preschooler serving).

SERVING SIZE

Toddler	1 toast stick
Preschooler	2 toast sticks
Adult	4 toast sticks

Nutrition Facts: Most of the nutrition facts labels in the recipes are based on a preschooler serving size.

Freezer Friendly: Recipes with the "Freezer Friendly" icon can be frozen, thawed and reheated at a later date.

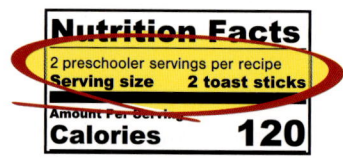
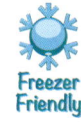

Kitchen safety

It is important to stay safe in the kitchen. Here are basic safety rules to follow in the kitchen:

1. A grown-up must be in the kitchen during all activities, including cooking and cleaning up.
2. Everyone must wash their hands with soap and water before touching food. If your child has long hair, it should be tied back. Roll shirt sleeves up, so they do not get wet or dirty.
3. Start with a clean kitchen. Wipe down countertops and put away things that you will not need.
4. Knives and sharp kitchen tools should be kept out of the reach of children and away from their working space.
5. Do not allow your child near a hot stove or oven. Keep pot handles pointed towards the center when they are placed on the stove.
6. Read the recipe out loud to your child and work slowly, doing one job at a time.

HAND WASHING

1. Get your hands wet and soapy with warm water.
2. Rub your soapy hands together and sing "Happy Birthday" twice. Be sure to clean everywhere on your hands: palms, back of your hands, fingers, and especially under your nails.
3. Rinse. Hold your hands under clean, running water. Rub them to rinse them fully.
4. Shake and dry. Shake your hands a few times, then dry them with a clean towel or hand dryer. **Done!**

Tip: If your child cannot reach the sink, hold them up to reach the sink. If your child can stand, use a safety step to boost them up to the faucet.

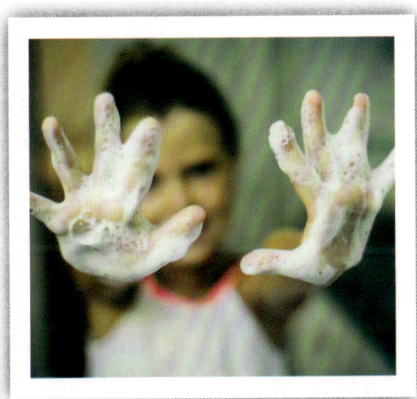

kitchen safety 25

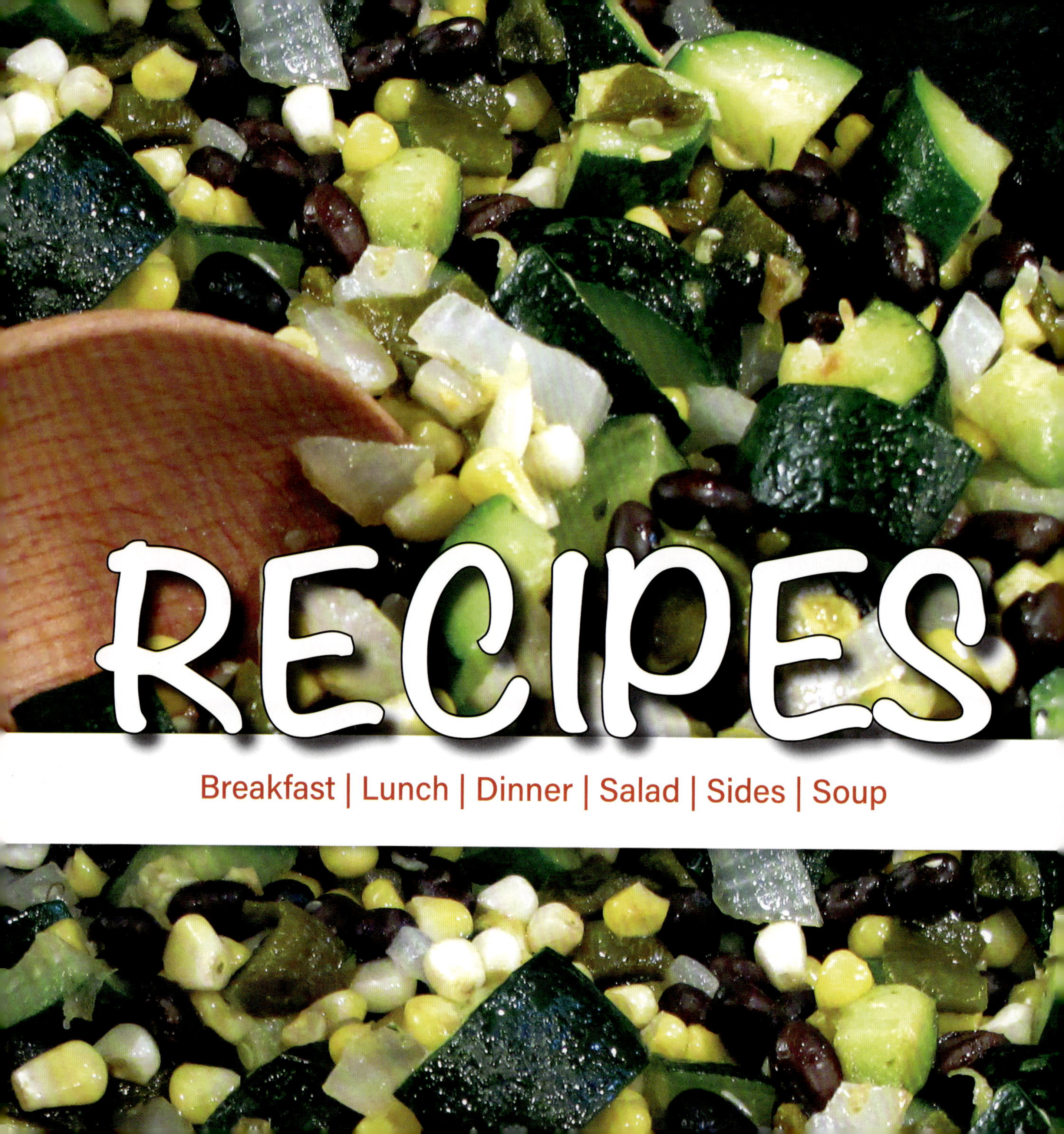

RECIPES

Breakfast | Lunch | Dinner | Salad | Sides | Soup

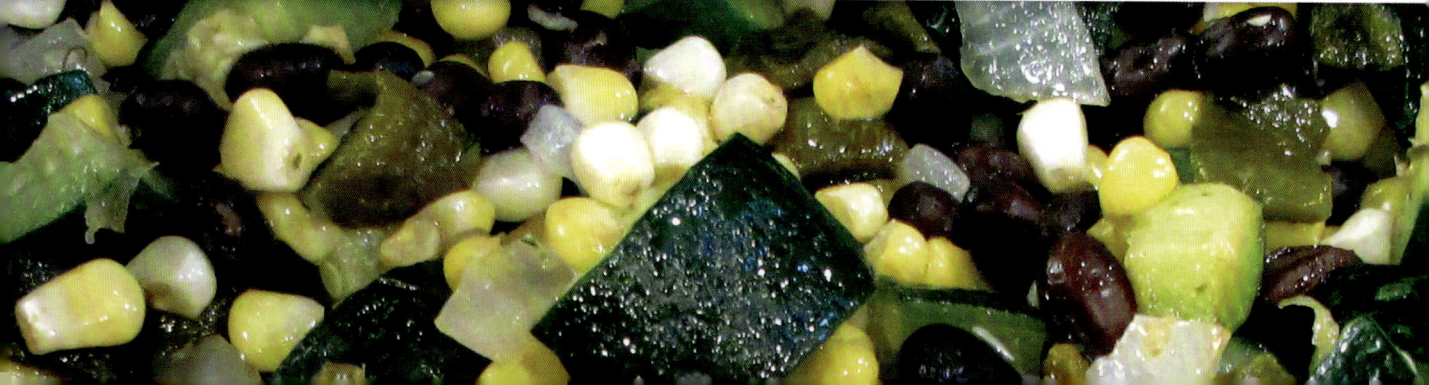

BREAKFAST

Avocado Toast Sticks 28
Best Ever Granola 29
Breakfast Burrito 30
No Bake Cereal Bars 31
PB&J Overnight Oatmeal 32
Pumpkin Pancakes 33
Smoothies 34

LUNCH

Egg Salad Sandwich 36
Hard-Boiled Eggs 36
Homemade Hummus. 37
Hummus Stuffed Pita Pockets. 37
Quesadilla 38
Peanut Butter & Banana Sushi Rolls . . 40
Salmon Salad 41
Salmon Salad Roll Ups 41
Savory Sunshine Wraps 42
Sweet Sunshine Wraps 42

DINNER

Chicken & Peas Mac n' Cheese 43
Classic Cheese Sauce 43
Creamy Pasta Primavera. 44
Green Chicken & Rice Bake. 45
Homemade Pizza 46
Parmesan Pork Sheet Pan Dinner 48
Pirate Planks. 49
Shroomy Stroganoff 50
Tuna Casserole. 51

SALAD

Avocado & Orange Salad 52
Cabbage Patch Slaw 52
Creamy "Cuke" Salad. 53
Sweet Tomato Salad. 53

SIDES

Calabecitas 54
Candied Peas & Carrots 54
Cauliflower Rice. 55
Cornbread 55
Crispy Kale. 56
Frosted Zucchini 56
Sand Castle Couscous. 57
Smashed Potatoes 57
Roasted Vegetables 58
Steamed Vegetables. 59

SOUP

Black Bean Soup. 60
Cream of Asparagus Soup 61
Creamy Cauliflower Soup. 62
Lentil Stew. 63
Wedding Soup 64

AVOCADO TOAST STICKS

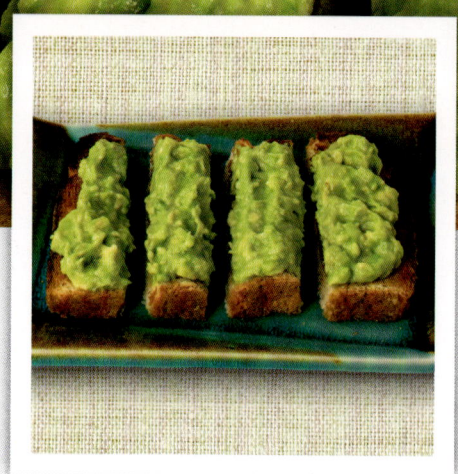

INGREDIENTS:
1 slice whole wheat bread
½ avocado, cut into 1-inch pieces
1 tsp lime juice
Pinch salt

DIRECTIONS:
1. Toast the bread.
2. Add avocado, lime juice and salt to a bowl and mash with a fork until mostly smooth.
3. Spread avocado mixture evenly on the toast.
4. Cut toast into 4 pieces. Serve. Makes 4 toast sticks.

SERVING SIZE

Toddler	1 toast stick
Preschooler	2 toast sticks
Adult	4 toast sticks

Nutrition Facts
2 preschooler servings per recipe
Serving size 2 toast sticks

Amount Per Serving
Calories 120

	% Daily Value*
Total Fat 8g	10%
Saturated Fat 1g	5%
Trans Fat 0g	
Cholesterol 0mg	0%
Sodium 140mg	6%
Total Carbohydrate 10g	4%
Dietary Fiber 4g	14%
Total Sugars <1g	
Incl. Added Sugars 0g	0%
Protein 3g	
Vitamin D 0mcg	0%
Calcium 30mg	2%
Iron 0.6mg	4%
Potassium 280mg	6%

* The % Daily Value (DV) tells you how much a nutrient in a serving of food contributes to a daily diet. 2,000 calories a day is used for general nutrition advice.

BEST EVER GRANOLA

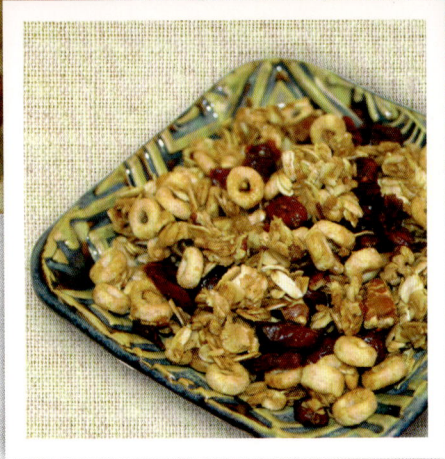

INGREDIENTS:

- 4 cups rolled oats
- 1 cup Cheerios™ (or other breakfast cereal)
- ½ cup chopped pecans or almonds
- ½ cup packed brown sugar
- ½ tsp salt
- ½ tsp cinnamon
- ¼ cup vegetable oil
- ¼ cup honey or maple syrup
- 1 tsp vanilla
- 1 cup raisins or dried cranberries

DIRECTIONS:

1. Preheat the oven to 300°F.
2. In a large bowl, mix the oats, Cheerios™, pecans, brown sugar, salt, and cinnamon.
3. In a saucepan, warm the oil and honey. Stir in the vanilla.
4. Carefully pour the liquid over the oat mixture and stir gently with a wooden spoon until evenly coated.
5. Spread the granola onto a large 15 x 10 x 1 inch cookie sheet. Bake 40 minutes, stirring carefully every 10 minutes. Remove from the oven and cool completely.
6. Stir in raisins or dried cranberries. Store in an air-tight container for 2 weeks. Makes 7 cups.

SERVING SIZE

Toddler	¼ cup
Preschooler	½ cup
Adult	1 cup

Nutrition Facts

14 preschooler servings per recipe

Serving size 1/2 cup

Amount Per Serving

Calories 240

	% Daily Value*
Total Fat 9g	12%
Saturated Fat 3.5g	18%
Trans Fat 0g	
Cholesterol 0mg	0%
Sodium 95mg	4%
Total Carbohydrate 40g	15%
Dietary Fiber 3g	11%
Total Sugars 20g	
Includes 13g Added Sugars	26%
Protein 4g	
Vitamin D 0.1mcg	0%
Calcium 20mg	2%
Iron 2.1mg	10%
Potassium 130mg	2%

*The % Daily Value (DV) tells you how much a nutrient in a serving of food contributes to a daily diet. 2,000 calories a day is used for general nutrition advice.

BREAKFAST BURRITO

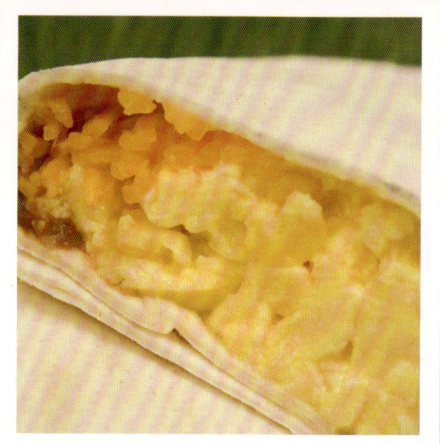

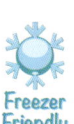
Freezer Friendly

INGREDIENTS:
- 1 egg
- ½ tsp water
- 1 Tbsp corn (frozen, canned or fresh)
- 1 (8-inch) whole wheat or flour tortilla
- 2 Tbsp shredded cheddar cheese
- 1 tsp medium salsa
- Non-stick cooking spray

DIRECTIONS:
1. Crack the egg into a small bowl. Add water. Using a fork, beat the egg until well mixed. Stir in the corn.
2. Heat a non-stick pan over medium heat. Spray with non-stick cooking spray.
3. Pour the egg mixture into the pan. Stir with a rubber spatula or a wooden spoon until the egg is cooked (about 2 minutes).
4. Place the egg in a line down the middle of the tortilla, sprinkle with cheese and salsa. Fold in the two sides of the tortilla and roll it up. Serve. Makes 1 burrito.

SERVING SIZE

Toddler	¼ burrito
Preschooler	½ burrito
Adult	1 burrito

Nutrition Facts

2 preschooler servings per recipe

Serving size 1/2 burrito

Amount Per Serving

Calories 130

	% Daily Value*
Total Fat 6g	8%
Saturated Fat 2g	10%
Trans Fat 0g	
Cholesterol 100mg	33%
Sodium 250mg	11%
Total Carbohydrate 13g	5%
Dietary Fiber 2g	7%
Total Sugars 0g	
Includes 0g Added Sugars	0%
Protein 7g	
Vitamin D 0.5mcg	2%
Calcium 110mg	8%
Iron 1mg	6%
Potassium 50mg	0%

* The % Daily Value (DV) tells you how much a nutrient in a serving of food contributes to a daily diet. 2,000 calories a day is used for general nutrition advice.

30 breakfast

NO BAKE CEREAL BARS

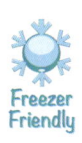
Freezer Friendly

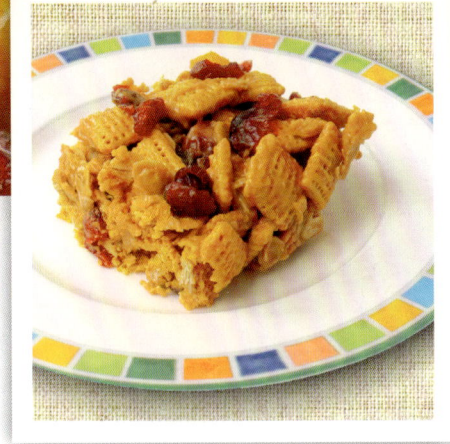

INGREDIENTS:

¾ cup peanut butter
¼ cup honey
2 Tbsp vegetable oil
3 cups Corn Chex™ (or other breakfast cereal)
1 cup rolled oats
¾ cup dried fruit (like raisins or apricots), chopped
Non-stick cooking spray

DIRECTIONS:

1. In a large pan, melt peanut butter, honey and oil.
2. Remove the pan from the heat and stir in Corn Chex™, oats and half of the dried fruit.
3. Spray an 8-inch square pan with non-stick cooking spray. Spread the mixture into the pan.
4. Sprinkle the rest of the dried fruit over top and press firmly.
5. Chill for 2 hours before cutting into bars. Store covered in the refrigerator for up to 2 weeks. Makes 9 bars.

SERVING SIZE

Toddler	¼ bar
Preschooler	½ bar
Adult	1 bar

Nutrition Facts

18 preschooler servings per recipe
Serving size 1/2 bar

Amount Per Serving
Calories 150

% Daily Value*

Total Fat 7g — 9%
Saturated Fat 2.5g — 13%
Trans Fat 0g
Cholesterol 0mg — 0%
Sodium 85mg — 4%
Total Carbohydrate 19g — 7%
Dietary Fiber 2g — 7%
Total Sugars 10g
Includes 4g Added Sugars — 8%
Protein 4g

Vitamin D 0.2mcg — 0%
Calcium 30mg — 2%
Iron 2.2mg — 10%
Potassium 70mg — 2%

* The % Daily Value (DV) tells you how much a nutrient in a serving of food contributes to a daily diet. 2,000 calories a day is used for general nutrition advice.

breakfast

PB&J OVERNIGHT OATMEAL

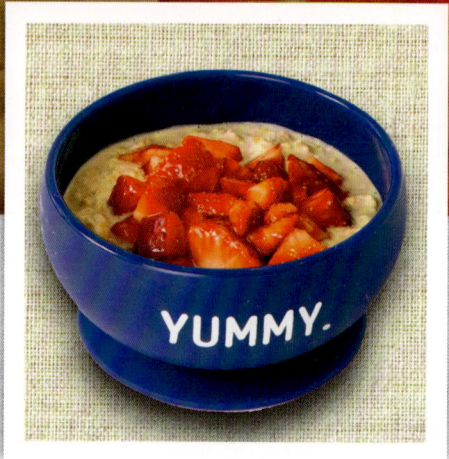

INGREDIENTS:

- 1 cup rolled oats
- 1 cup 2% low-fat milk
- 2 Tbsp peanut butter
- 4 strawberries, diced
- 1 tsp jelly, any flavor

DIRECTIONS:

1. Add oats, milk and peanut butter to a jar or container with a lid.
2. Cover the container and refrigerate overnight.
3. In the morning, remove the lid from the container.
4. Gently mix the strawberries and jelly together and spoon the fruit mixture over the oatmeal. Enjoy cold. Store in refrigerator for 2 days. Makes 2 cups.

SERVING SIZE

Toddler	¼ cup
Preschooler	½ cup
Adult	1 cup

Nutrition Facts

4 preschooler servings per recipe

Serving size 1/2 cup

Amount Per Serving

Calories 170

	% Daily Value*
Total Fat 7g	9%
Saturated Fat 2g	10%
Trans Fat 0g	
Cholesterol <5mg	2%
Sodium 70mg	3%
Total Carbohydrate 21g	8%
Dietary Fiber 3g	11%
Total Sugars 6g	
Includes 1g Added Sugars	2%
Protein 7g	
Vitamin D 0.6mcg	4%
Calcium 90mg	8%
Iron 1.1mg	6%
Potassium 180mg	4%

* The % Daily Value (DV) tells you how much a nutrient in a serving of food contributes to a daily diet. 2,000 calories a day is used for general nutrition advice.

breakfast

PUMPKIN PANCAKES

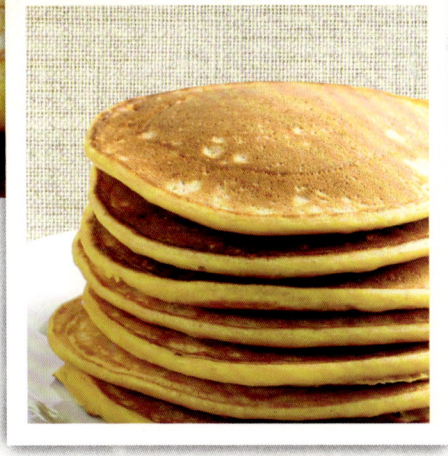

INGREDIENTS:

2 cups pancake mix
1 cup 2% low-fat milk
1 egg
½ cup canned pumpkin puree
2 Tbsp sugar
½ tsp ground cinnamon
Non-stick cooking spray

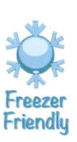
Freezer Friendly

DIRECTIONS:

1. In a medium/large bowl, combine all the ingredients until just blended (batter can be a little lumpy).
2. Spray skillet pan with non-stick cooking spray and heat over medium heat. Spoon ¼ cup of batter into pan to form each pancake. Cook until edges are drying and bubbles start to pop.
3. Using a flat spatula, flip each pancake and cook 2-3 minutes longer.
4. Serve with maple syrup and banana slices. Makes 12 pancakes.

SERVING SIZE

Toddler	1 pancake
Preschooler	2 pancakes
Adult	3 pancakes

Nutrition Facts
6 preschooler servings per recipe
Serving size: 2 pancakes

Amount Per Serving
Calories 190

% Daily Value*

Total Fat 2.5g	3%
Saturated Fat 0.5g	3%
Trans Fat 0g	
Cholesterol 30mg	10%
Sodium 340mg	15%
Total Carbohydrate 36g	13%
Dietary Fiber 8g	29%
Total Sugars 8g	
Includes 4g Added Sugars	8%
Protein 8g	
Vitamin D 0.6mcg	2%
Calcium 120mg	10%
Iron 2.7mg	15%
Potassium 90mg	2%

* The % Daily Value (DV) tells you how much a nutrient in a serving of food contributes to a daily diet. 2,000 calories a day is used for general nutrition advice.

breakfast

SMOOTHIES

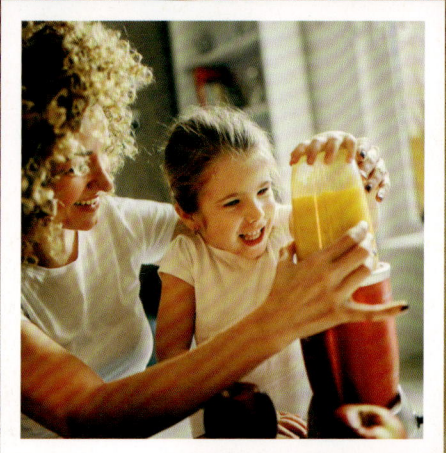

Smoothies are easy and quick to make. You can prepare them in advance and they're great on the go.

Combine a variety of fruits and/or vegetables. A few smoothie recipe ideas are listed here but the options are endless!

INGREDIENTS:

Fruits or Veggies: 2 – 3 cups
fresh, frozen or canned (in 100% juice or water)

Liquid: 1 – 1 ½ cups
2% low-fat or skim milk, 100% juice, yogurt, or ice cubes

Extras (optional): 1 – 2 Tbsp
peanut butter, ground nuts, wheat germ or honey

DIRECTIONS:

Add ingredients to a blender and blend until smooth. Pour into a glass and enjoy.

Each recipe makes about three 6-ounce servings.

	FRUITS OR VEGGIES	LIQUID
Banana Berry	1 banana, peeled and broken into 4 pieces 3 strawberries	½ cup 100% apple juice ½ cup 2% low-fat milk
Blueberry Avocado	½ banana, peeled and broken into 2 pieces 1 cup blueberries ½ avocado, pitted and cut into 4 chunks	½ cup 100% apple juice ½ cup 2% low-fat milk 1 Tbsp lemon juice
Peach Spinach	1 banana, peeled and broken into 4 pieces 1 cup peaches ½ cup spinach	1 cup 2% low-fat milk
Mango Carrot	½ banana, peeled and broken into 2 pieces 3 baby carrots 1 cup mango chunks	1 cup 2% low-fat milk

breakfast

EGG SALAD SANDWICH

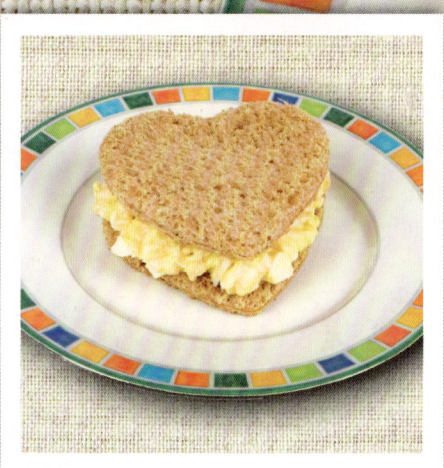

INGREDIENTS:
- 2 hard-boiled eggs, peeled (recipe below)
- 1 Tbsp of mayonnaise
- 2 slices whole wheat bread

DIRECTIONS:
1. Chop the eggs and place them in a small mixing bowl.
2. Mix with mayonnaise.
3. Spread egg salad on bread to make a sandwich. Store leftover egg salad in the refrigerator for 2 days. Makes 1 sandwich.

HARD-BOILED EGGS

DIRECTIONS:
1. Place 8 eggs in a large pot and add enough cold water to cover the eggs. Cook on high heat until the water starts to boil. Once water boils, cover the pan and turn off heat.
2. Let the eggs stand for 20 minutes. Place eggs in a bowl of ice water and allow the eggs to cool.
3. Using a marker or pencil, mark each egg with the date. Store hard-boiled eggs (in the shell) for up to one week in the refrigerator.

Simply peel the shell from the egg before eating.

SERVING SIZE

Toddler	¼ sandwich
Preschooler	½ sandwich
Adult	1 sandwich

Nutrition Facts

2 preschooler servings per recipe
Serving size 1/2 sandwich

Amount Per Serving
Calories 190

	% Daily Value*
Total Fat 11g	14%
Saturated Fat 2.5g	13%
Trans Fat 0g	
Cholesterol 190mg	63%
Sodium 230mg	10%
Total Carbohydrate 13g	5%
Dietary Fiber 2g	7%
Total Sugars 2g	
Includes 0g Added Sugars	0%
Protein 10g	
Vitamin D 1.1mcg	6%
Calcium 70mg	6%
Iron 1.3mg	8%
Potassium 140mg	2%

* The % Daily Value (DV) tells you how much a nutrient in a serving of food contributes to a daily diet. 2,000 calories a day is used for general nutrition advice.

HUMMUS STUFFED PITA POCKETS

INGREDIENTS:
- ¼ cucumber, diced
- 2 cherry tomatoes, diced
- ½ cup lettuce, shredded
- ¼ cup hummus (recipe below or store-bought)
- 1 whole wheat pita bread

DIRECTIONS:
1. Cut pita in half. Using a knife, open a pocket on each half. Spread the hummus inside both pita pockets.
2. Stuff the pockets with shredded lettuce, cucumber and tomato. Makes 2 pita pockets.

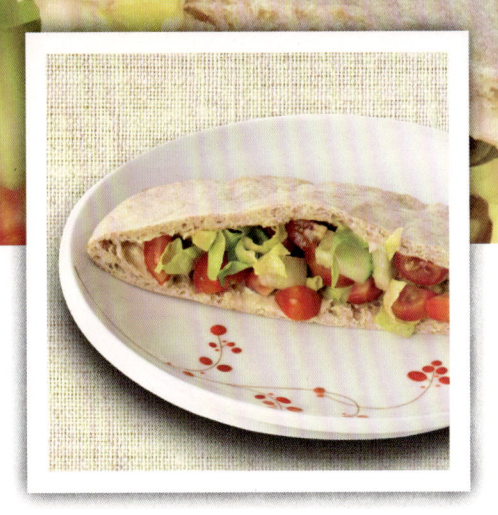

SERVING SIZE

Toddler	½ pita pocket
Preschooler	1 pita pocket
Adult	2 pita pockets

HOMEMADE HUMMUS

INGREDIENTS:
- 1 can (15 oz.) chickpeas (garbanzo beans), rinsed and drained
- 1 garlic clove, peeled and chopped
- 2 Tbsp smooth peanut butter
- 2 Tbsp vegetable oil
- 2 Tbsp lemon juice (about 1 lemon)
- ¼ cup water

DIRECTIONS:
Place all ingredients in a blender and process until smooth. If needed, add 1-2 Tablespoons more water for a creamy texture. Refrigerate in a covered container for 5-7 days. Makes 1 ½ cups.

Nutrition Facts

2 preschooler servings per recipe
Serving size 1 pita pocket

Amount Per Serving
Calories 150

	% Daily Value*
Total Fat 3.5g	4%
Saturated Fat 0g	0%
Trans Fat 0g	
Cholesterol 0mg	0%
Sodium 290mg	13%
Total Carbohydrate 24g	9%
Dietary Fiber 5g	18%
Total Sugars 3g	
Includes 0g Added Sugars	0%
Protein 6g	
Vitamin D 0mcg	0%
Calcium 30mg	2%
Iron 1.9mg	10%
Potassium 180mg	4%

* The % Daily Value (DV) tells you how much a nutrient in a serving of food contributes to a daily diet. 2,000 calories a day is used for general nutrition advice.

QUESADILLA

SERVING SIZE

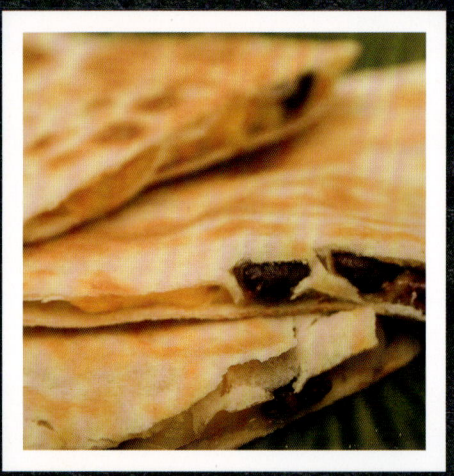

Toddler	¼ quesadilla
Preschooler	½ quesadilla
Adult	1 quesadilla

Nutrition Facts

2 preschooler servings per recipe
Serving size 1/2 quesadilla

Amount Per Serving
Calories 330

	% Daily Value*
Total Fat 15g	19%
Saturated Fat 8g	40%
Trans Fat 0g	
Cholesterol 15mg	5%
Sodium 560mg	24%
Total Carbohydrate 40g	15%
Dietary Fiber 3g	11%
Total Sugars 1g	
Includes 0g Added Sugars	0%
Protein 10g	
Vitamin D 0mcg	0%
Calcium 200mg	15%
Iron 2.6mg	15%
Potassium 160mg	4%

* The % Daily Value (DV) tells you how much a nutrient in a serving of food contributes to a daily diet. 2,000 calories a day is used for general nutrition advice.

INGREDIENTS:
- 2 Tbsp black beans, rinsed and drained
- 1 Tbsp corn kernels
- ¼ cup shredded cheddar cheese
- 2 (8-inch) whole wheat or flour tortillas
- 2 tsp vegetable oil

Freezer Friendly

DIRECTIONS:
1. Place tortilla on a large plate and brush with oil. Flip it over. Sprinkle cheese, beans and corn over the tortilla.
2. Leave a ½-inch edge empty all the way around the tortilla. Place the other tortilla on top of the cheese mixture, making a sandwich.
3. Brush the top of the tortilla lightly with oil. Place the tortilla sandwich in a non-stick frying pan over medium heat.
4. Using a spatula, flip the tortilla when it is golden brown (about 2 minutes).
5. Brown the other side (about 2 minutes). Remove from pan and slice into pieces like a pie.

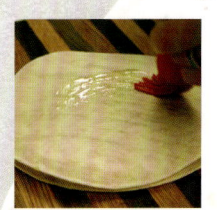

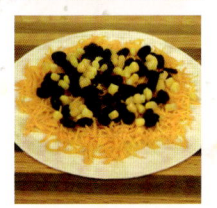

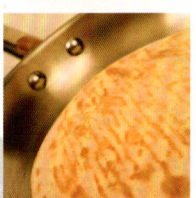

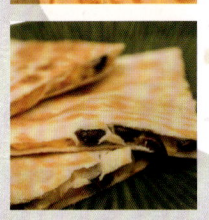

OTHER FILLINGS:

Quesadillas can be made with many foods. They are a terrific way to use leftovers.

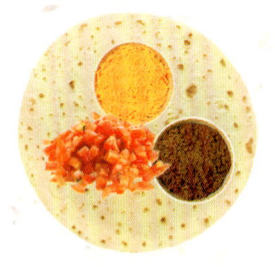

Taco meat,
chopped tomatoes and
shredded cheddar cheese

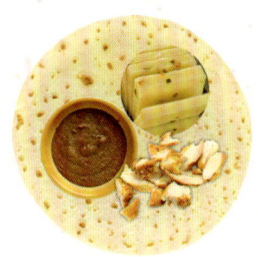

Grilled chicken,
refried beans and
shredded jack cheese

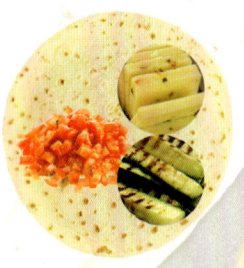

Grilled zucchini,
diced tomatoes and
shredded mozzarella cheese

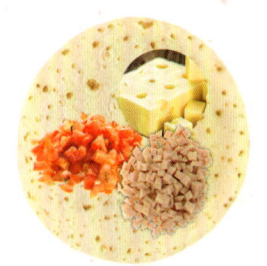

Deli-ham cut in squares,
diced tomatoes and
shredded Swiss cheese

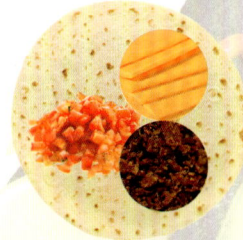

Bacon crumbles,
diced tomatoes and
American cheese

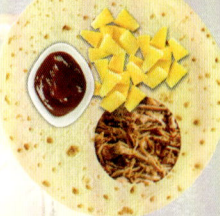

Pulled pork,
pineapple, bbq sauce and
shredded jack cheese

PEANUT BUTTER & BANANA SUSHI ROLLS

INGREDIENTS:

2 Tbsp peanut butter
1 small ripe banana, peeled
1 (8-inch) whole wheat or flour tortilla

DIRECTIONS:

1. Cut the edges off 2 sides of the tortilla.
2. Spread peanut butter over the tortilla.
3. Place the banana on top of the peanut butter, along the edge closest to you.
4. Fold the edge of the tortilla up and over the banana, keep rolling the tortilla around the banana. Cut into 5-6 even pieces. Makes 2 preschooler servings.

TIP: If the tortilla is dry, it will be difficult to roll up. To fix this problem, put the tortilla between 2 damp paper towels and microwave on HIGH for 10 seconds.

SERVING SIZE

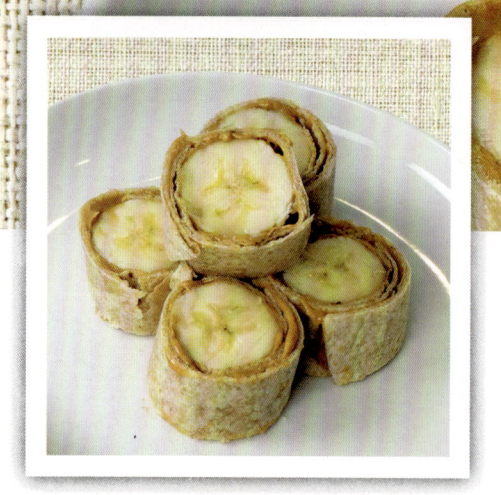

Toddler	1–2 pieces
Preschooler	2–3 pieces
Adult	5–6 pieces

Nutrition Facts

2 preschooler servings per recipe
Serving size 1/2 recipe

Amount Per Serving
Calories 200

	% Daily Value*
Total Fat 10g	13%
Saturated Fat 1.5g	8%
Trans Fat 0g	
Cholesterol 0mg	0%
Sodium 230mg	10%
Total Carbohydrate 26g	9%
Dietary Fiber 4g	14%
Total Sugars 8g	
Includes 0g Added Sugars	0%
Protein 6g	
Vitamin D 0mcg	0%
Calcium 60mcg	4%
Iron 0.9mg	6%
Potassium 270mg	6%

* The % Daily Value (DV) tells you how much a nutrient in a serving of food contributes to a daily diet. 2,000 calories a day is used for general nutrition advice.

SALMON SALAD ROLL UPS

INGREDIENTS:

- 2 Tbsp salmon salad (recipe below)
- 1 steamed green bean
- 1 slice whole wheat bread, crust removed

DIRECTIONS:

1. Spread 2 tablespoons of salmon salad evenly on the bread.
2. Place the bean on one side of the bread and roll it up from one side to the other. Slice in half and serve. Makes 2 roll ups.

SALMON SALAD

INGREDIENTS:

- 1 can (7.5 oz) pink salmon
- 4 oz cream cheese
- 1 Tbsp 2% low-fat milk

DIRECTIONS:

1. In a small bowl mix together all ingredients. This recipe makes enough salmon salad for 12 roll ups.
2. Refrigerate in a covered container for 2-3 days.

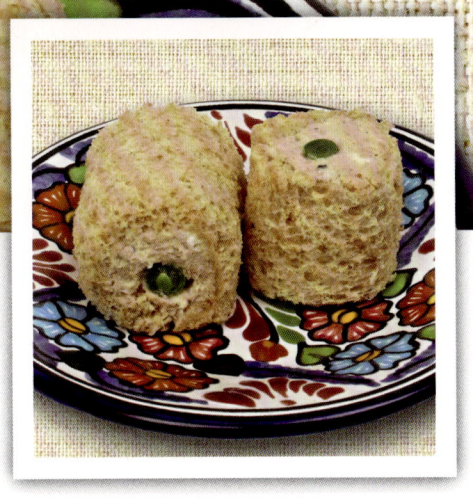

SERVING SIZE

Toddler	1 roll up
Preschooler	2 roll ups
Adult	4 roll ups

Nutrition Facts

1 preschooler serving per recipe
Serving size: 2 roll ups

Amount Per Serving
Calories 230

% Daily Value*

Total Fat 11g	14%
Saturated Fat 4.5g	23%
Trans Fat 0g	
Cholesterol 55mg	18%
Sodium 460mg	20%
Total Carbohydrate 14g	5%
Dietary Fiber 2g	7%
Total Sugars 2g	
Includes 0g Added Sugars	0%
Protein 18g	
Vitamin D 9.4mcg	45%
Calcium 220mg	15%
Iron 1.2mg	6%
Potassium 350mg	8%

* The % Daily Value (DV) tells you how much a nutrient in a serving of food contributes to a daily diet. 2,000 calories a day is used for general nutrition advice.

lunch

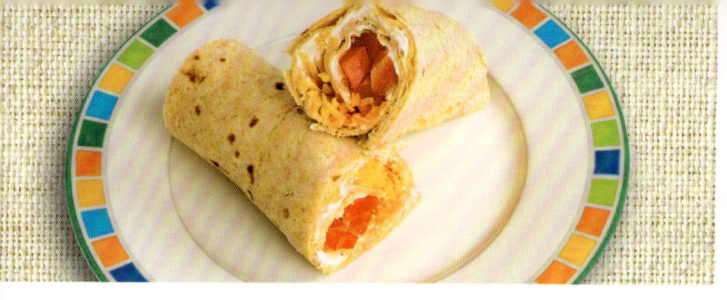

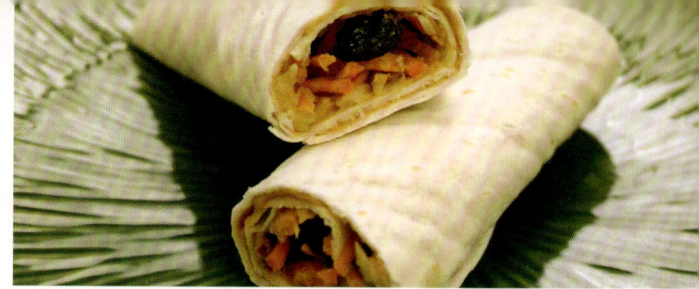

SAVORY SUNSHINE WRAPS

INGREDIENTS:
2 Tbsp cream cheese
1 Tbsp shredded cheddar cheese
1 Tbsp carrots, shredded
1 Tbsp red bell pepper, diced
1 (8-inch) whole wheat or flour tortilla

DIRECTIONS:
1. Spread cream cheese over the tortilla.
2. Sprinkle half of the tortilla with carrots, red peppers and cheese.
3. Beginning on the side with the carrot mixture, roll up the tortilla. The cream cheese will act like glue to seal the wrap. Serve. Makes 1 wrap or 2 preschooler servings.

Nutrition Facts Servings: 2, Serv. Size: 1/2
Amount Per Recipe : **Calories 130, Total Fat** 8g (10% DV), Sat. Fat 3.5g (18% DV), *Trans* Fat 0g, **Cholest.** 20mg (7% DV), **Sodium** 230mg (10% DV), **Total Carb.** 13g (5% DV), Fiber 2g (7% DV), Total Sugars <1g (Incl. 0g Added Sugars, 0% DV), **Protein** 4g, Vit. D (0% DV), Calcium (6% DV), Iron (4% DV), Potas. (0% DV).

SWEET SUNSHINE WRAPS

INGREDIENTS:
2 Tbsp peanut butter
1 Tbsp apple, shredded
1 Tbsp carrots, shredded
8-10 raisins
1 (8-inch) whole wheat or flour tortilla

DIRECTIONS:
1. Spread peanut butter over the tortilla.
2. Sprinkle half of the tortilla with carrots, apple, and raisins.
3. Beginning on the side with the carrot mixture, roll up the tortilla. The peanut butter will act like glue to seal the wrap. Serve. Makes 1 wrap or 2 preschooler servings.

Nutrition Facts Servings: 2, Serv. Size: 1/2
Amount Per Recipe : **Calories 170, Total Fat** 10g (13% DV), Sat. Fat 2g (10% DV), *Trans* Fat 0g, **Cholest.** 0mg (0% DV), **Sodium** 230mg (10% DV), **Total Carb.** 18g (7% DV), Fiber 2g (7% DV), Total Sugars 3g (Incl. <1g Added Sugars, 1% DV), **Protein** 6g, Vit. D (0% DV), Calcium (4% DV), Iron (6% DV), Potas. (4% DV).

CHICKEN & PEAS MAC N' CHEESE

INGREDIENTS:
- Classic Cheese Sauce (recipe below)
- 2 cups dry elbow macaroni
- ½ cup frozen peas
- ½ cup cooked chicken, cubed or shredded

DIRECTIONS:
1. Make Classic Cheese Sauce (recipe below).
2. Cook peas and macaroni, according to the package directions. Drain in a colander and return to the pan.
3. Over low heat, add the cooked chicken and cheese sauce. Toss gently to coat the macaroni with sauce. Makes 5 adult or 10 preschooler servings.

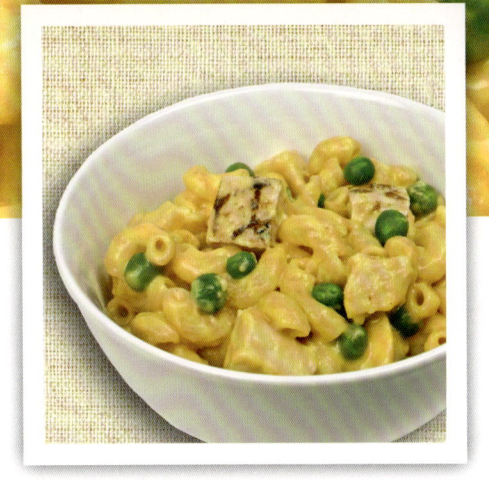

Freezer Friendly

SERVING SIZE

Toddler	¼ cup
Preschooler	½ cup
Adult	1 cup

CLASSIC CHEESE SAUCE

INGREDIENTS:
- 2 Tbsp of butter or margarine
- 2 Tbsp flour
- 1 ½ cups 2% low-fat milk
- 1 ½ cups shredded cheddar cheese

DIRECTIONS:
1. In a saucepan melt butter over medium heat. Stir in flour and cook for 2 minutes.
2. Continue to stir and SLOWLY pour in the milk. Add the cheese. Continue to stir until melted.

Nutrition Facts
10 preschooler servings per recipe
Serving size: 1/2 cup

Amount Per Serving
Calories 210

	% Daily Value*
Total Fat 9g	12%
Saturated Fat 5g	25%
Trans Fat 0g	
Cholesterol 35mg	12%
Sodium 160mg	7%
Total Carbohydrate 20g	7%
Dietary Fiber 1g	4%
Total Sugars 3g	
Includes 0g Added Sugars	0%
Protein 11g	
Vitamin D 0.4mcg	2%
Calcium 180mg	15%
Iron 1mg	6%
Potassium 140mg	4%

* The % Daily Value (DV) tells you how much a nutrient in a serving of food contributes to a daily diet. 2,000 calories a day is used for general nutrition advice.

dinner 43

CREAMY PASTA PRIMAVERA

INGREDIENTS:

3 cups dry spiral (rotini) pasta
1 cup asparagus, trimmed and cut in 2-inch pieces
½ cup red pepper, diced
1 small yellow summer squash, cut into thin circles
5 baby carrots, cut into thin strips
4 oz. cream cheese, cubed
½ cup grated parmesan cheese
2 Tbsp lemon juice

Freezer Friendly

DIRECTIONS:

1. Cook the pasta according to the package directions. During the last 3 minutes of cooking, add the asparagus, bell peppers, zucchini and carrots to the boiling water. Pour ½ cup of pasta water into a measuring cup. Drain the pasta and vegetables into a colander.

2. In the same pot, add the pasta water, cream cheese, parmesan cheese, and lemon juice. Stir over low heat until the cheese is melted. Add the pasta and vegetables. Gently toss with sauce. Makes 6 adult or 12 preschooler servings.

TIP: Using flavored cream cheese, such as garlic herb, instead of plain cream cheese, will add additional flavor to this recipe.

SERVING SIZE

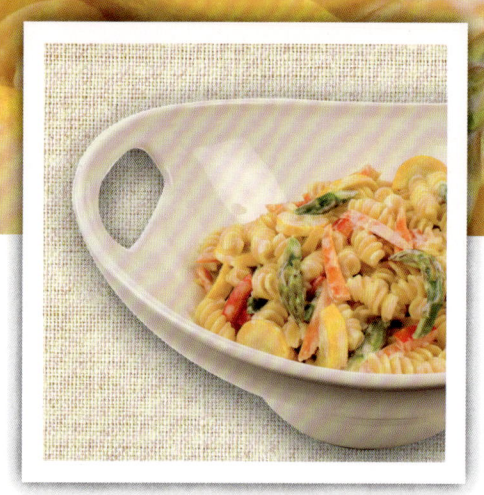

Toddler	¼ cup
Preschooler	½ cup
Adult	1 cup

Nutrition Facts

12 preschooler servings per recipe
Serving size 1/2 cup

Amount Per Serving
Calories 150

	% Daily Value*
Total Fat 7g	9%
Saturated Fat 4.5g	23%
Trans Fat 0g	
Cholesterol 15mg	5%
Sodium 110mg	5%
Total Carbohydrate 17g	6%
Dietary Fiber 1g	4%
Total Sugars 2g	
Includes 0g Added Sugars	0%
Protein 5g	
Vitamin D 0mcg	0%
Calcium 50mg	4%
Iron 1mg	6%
Potassium 140mg	2%

* The % Daily Value (DV) tells you how much a nutrient in a serving of food contributes to a daily diet. 2,000 calories a day is used for general nutrition advice.

dinner

GREEN CHICKEN & RICE BAKE

INGREDIENTS:

- 1 package (12 oz.) frozen broccoli florets
- 1 cup dry brown or white rice
- ¾ cup low sodium chicken broth
- ¼ cup mayonnaise
- 1 tsp salt
- 2 Tbsp lemon juice
- ¾ cup 2% low-fat milk
- 2 cups cooked chicken, diced
- ¾ cup shredded cheddar cheese

Freezer Friendly

DIRECTIONS:

1. Preheat the oven to 350°F. Cook broccoli and rice according to the package directions.
2. Place the cooked broccoli, chicken broth, mayonnaise, salt and lemon juice in a blender. Process to a smooth puree.
3. In an oven-proof casserole dish, add the rice, milk, chicken and ½ cup of cheese. Pour the broccoli mixture over the top. Toss the mixture gently to blend ingredients.
4. Place in the oven for 15-20 minutes or until heated through and the cheese is melted. Makes 6 adult or 12 preschooler servings.

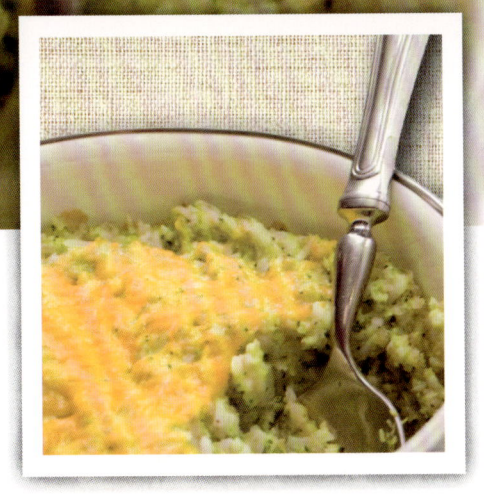

SERVING SIZE

Toddler	¼ cup
Preschooler	½ cup
Adult	1 cup

Nutrition Facts

12 preschooler servings per recipe

Serving size 1/2 cup

Amount Per Serving

Calories 170

	% Daily Value*
Total Fat 7g	9%
Saturated Fat 2.5g	13%
Trans Fat 0g	
Cholesterol 30mg	10%
Sodium 310mg	13%
Total Carbohydrate 15g	5%
Dietary Fiber 1g	4%
Total Sugars 1g	
Includes 0g Added Sugars	0%
Protein 12g	
Vitamin D 0.2mcg	0%
Calcium 100mg	8%
Iron 0.6mg	4%
Potassium 190mg	4%

* The % Daily Value (DV) tells you how much a nutrient in a serving of food contributes to a daily diet. 2,000 calories a day is used for general nutrition advice.

HOMEMADE PIZZA

INGREDIENTS:
1 ready-to-bake pizza dough (like Pillsbury™)
1 cup pasta sauce
1 cup shredded part-skim mozzarella cheese
Non-stick cooking spray

Freezer Friendly

DIRECTIONS:
1. Preheat oven to 400°F. Spray a 13 x 9 x 2-inch pan with non-stick cooking spray.
2. Open the dough. Place it evenly over the bottom of the pan.
3. Spread the pasta sauce evenly over the dough.
4. Leave a ½-inch edge without sauce on all 4 sides of the dough. Sprinkle the cheese over the sauce.
5. Add toppings (see below) and bake for 12-14 minutes. Let stand 3 minutes before cutting into slices. Store leftovers in the refrigerator for up to 3 days. Makes 8 slices.

SERVING SIZE

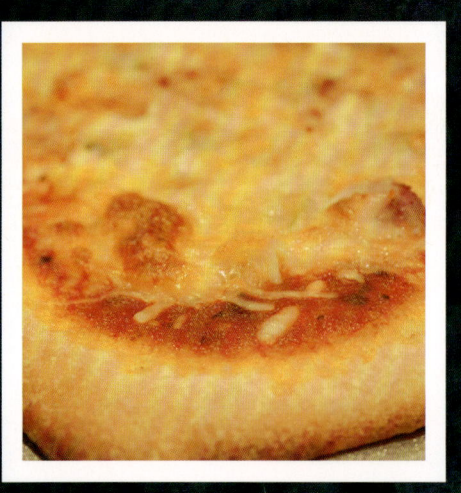

Toddler	1 slice
Preschooler	2 slices
Adult	4 slices

Nutrition Facts
4 preschooler servings per recipe
Serving size   **2 slices**

Amount Per Serving
Calories   **220**

	% Daily Value*
Total Fat 4g	5%
Saturated Fat 1.5g	8%
Trans Fat 0g	
Cholesterol 10mg	3%
Sodium 530mg	23%
Total Carbohydrate 37g	13%
Dietary Fiber 2g	7%
Total Sugars 3g	
Includes 2g Added Sugars	4%
Protein 9g	
Vitamin D 0mcg	0%
Calcium 120mg	10%
Iron 2.5mg	15%
Potassium 120mg	2%

* The % Daily Value (DV) tells you how much a nutrient in a serving of food contributes to a daily diet. 2,000 calories a day is used for general nutrition advice.

TOPPING IDEAS:

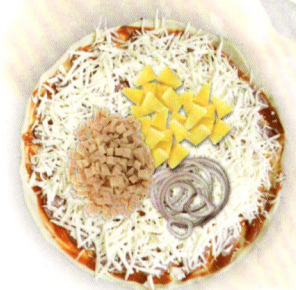

Hawaiian
ham, pineapple and thin-sliced red onion

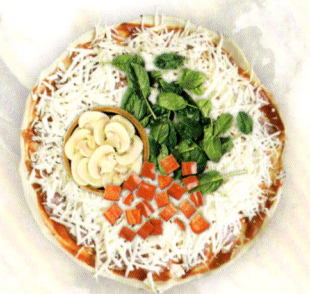

Veggie
spinach, sliced mushrooms and diced red pepper

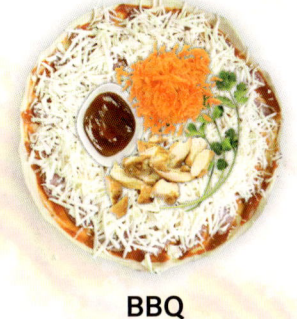

BBQ
replace pasta sauce with BBQ sauce, top with diced cooked chicken and shredded carrots. Sprinkle with chopped cilantro after cooking.

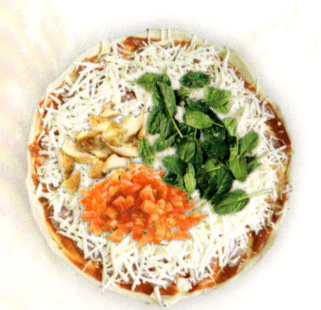

Mediterranean
diced tomatoes, chopped garlic, spinach and diced or shredded cooked chicken

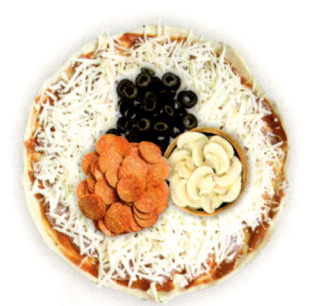

Italian
pepperoni, black olives and sliced mushrooms

PARMESAN PORK SHEET PAN DINNER

SERVING SIZE

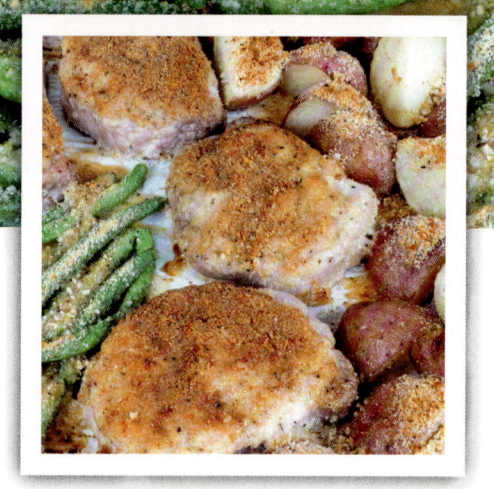

Toddler	¼ pork chop & veggies
Preschooler	½ pork chop & veggies
Adult	1 pork chop & veggies

INGREDIENTS:

- 1 lb. (7-9 small) red potatoes, quartered
- 3 Tbsp vegetable oil
- 4 boneless pork chops, ½-inch thick
- ½ cup grated parmesan cheese
- ½ cup breadcrumbs
- 1 tsp garlic powder
- ½ tsp black pepper
- 1 lb. green beans, ends trimmed

Freezer Friendly

DIRECTIONS:

1. Preheat oven to 375°F. Spray a large baking sheet with non-stick cooking spray.
2. Put the potatoes and 1 tablespoon oil in a bowl. Toss to coat the potatoes with oil. Spread the potatoes on one side of the baking sheet in a single layer.
3. Place the pork chops on the open side of the baking sheet. Rub the top of the pork chops with 1 tablespoon oil.
4. In a small bowl, mix the parmesan cheese, breadcrumbs, garlic powder, and black pepper. Spoon half of the mixture evenly over the pork chops. Press the mixture onto the pork chops. Bake for 20 minutes.
5. In a bowl, toss green beans with 1 tablespoon oil.
6. Remove the baking sheet from the oven and use a spatula to make room for the green beans. Sprinkle the remaining parmesan mixture over the potatoes and green beans. Bake for 15 minutes. Makes 4 adult or 8 preschooler servings.

Nutrition Facts

8 preschooler servings per recipe
Serving size 1/8 recipe

Amount Per Serving
Calories 230

	% Daily Value*
Total Fat 11g	14%
Saturated Fat 6g	30%
Trans Fat 0g	
Cholesterol 35mg	12%
Sodium 180mg	8%
Total Carbohydrate 15g	5%
Dietary Fiber 3g	11%
Total Sugars 3g	
Includes 0g Added Sugars	0%
Protein 18g	
Vitamin D 0.4mcg	2%
Calcium 80mg	6%
Iron 1.5mg	8%
Potassium 630mg	15%

* The % Daily Value (DV) tells you how much a nutrient in a serving of food contributes to a daily diet. 2,000 calories a day is used for general nutrition advice.

PIRATE PLANKS

INGREDIENTS:
- 2 tilapia fillets
- Dash of salt and pepper
- 1 egg
- 2 Tbsp cornmeal
- 2 Tbsp flour
- 2 Tbsp vegetable oil

DIRECTIONS:
1. Cut fish into strips about 1-inch wide and 3 inches long. Sprinkle fish with salt and pepper.
2. Crack the egg into a wide bowl and beat with a fork.
3. On a shallow plate mix the cornmeal and flour together.
4. Dip the fish pieces in egg and then coat both sides with the flour mixture.
5. Heat oil in a non-stick pan over medium heat. Place coated fish strips in the pan and cook, about 3 minutes. Flip the fish over and cook another 2-3 minutes. The fish should be nicely browned on both sides. Transfer fish to a paper towel. Makes about 8 fish sticks.

Serve fish sticks warm with a seafood dipping sauce (below).

SIMPLE SEAFOOD DIPPING SAUCES:
Tartar: Mayonnaise mixed with sweet pickle relish
Cocktail: Ketchup mixed with horseradish and lemon juice
Siracha Spicy Mayo: Mayonnaise mixed with siracha sauce

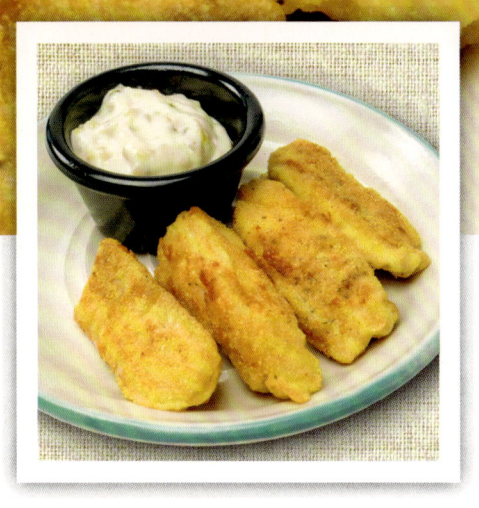

SERVING SIZE

Toddler	1 fish stick
Preschooler	2 fish sticks
Adult	4 fish sticks

Nutrition Facts
4 preschooler servings per recipe
Serving size 2 fish sticks

Amount Per Serving
Calories 190

	% Daily Value*
Total Fat 9g	12%
Saturated Fat 6g	30%
Trans Fat 0g	
Cholesterol 85mg	28%
Sodium 100mg	4%
Total Carbohydrate 7g	3%
Dietary Fiber 0g	0%
Total Sugars 0g	
Includes 0g Added Sugars	0%
Protein 19g	
Vitamin D 2.9mcg	15%
Calcium 20mg	2%
Iron 1mg	6%
Potassium 280mg	6%

* The % Daily Value (DV) tells you how much a nutrient in a serving of food contributes to a daily diet. 2,000 calories a day is used for general nutrition advice.

dinner

SHROOMY STROGANOFF

INGREDIENTS:

- 4 cups dry egg noodles
- 2 Tbsp butter or margarine
- ½ medium onion, diced
- 1 lb. fresh white mushrooms, sliced
- ½ cup low-sodium beef broth
- ½ tsp dried dill
- 1 cup sour cream

DIRECTIONS:

1. Prepare the egg noodles according to the package directions. Drain in a colander. Return noodles to the pan and cover to keep warm.
2. Melt the butter in a large skillet over medium-high heat. Add the onions and mushrooms and stir constantly for about 5 minutes.
3. Turn the heat to low and add the beef broth and dill. Continue cooking about 4 more minutes.
4. Add the sour cream. Gently stir until heated through, but do not allow it to boil.
5. To serve, spoon mushroom mixture over cooked egg noodles. Makes 4 adult or 8 preschooler servings.

SERVING SIZE

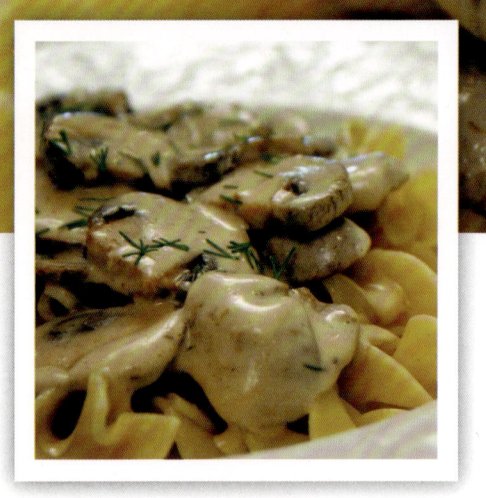

Toddler	¼ cup
Preschooler	½ cup
Adult	1 cup

Nutrition Facts

8 preschooler servings per recipe

Serving size 1/2 cup

Amount Per Serving

Calories 170

	% Daily Value*
Total Fat 10g	13%
Saturated Fat 5g	25%
Trans Fat 0g	
Cholesterol 40mg	13%
Sodium 95mg	4%
Total Carbohydrate 17g	6%
Dietary Fiber 1g	4%
Total Sugars 3g	
Includes 0g Added Sugars	0%
Protein 5g	
Vitamin D 0.2mcg	0%
Calcium 40mg	4%
Iron 1.1mg	6%
Potassium 280mg	6%

* The % Daily Value (DV) tells you how much a nutrient in a serving of food contributes to a daily diet. 2,000 calories a day is used for general nutrition advice.

TUNA CASSEROLE

INGREDIENTS:

- 3 cups dry egg noodles
- 1 yellow onion, minced
- 2 Tbsp butter or margarine
- ½ cup sliced mushrooms
- ½ cup frozen green peas
- 1 can cream of celery soup
- ¾ cup 2% low-fat milk
- 1 (5-oz.) can tuna in water, drained
- ¼ cup breadcrumbs
- Non-stick cooking spray

Freezer Friendly

DIRECTIONS:

1. Preheat the oven to 350°F. Spray an oven-proof casserole dish with cooking spray.
2. Cook the egg noodles according to the package directions. Drain in a colander and set aside.
3. In a large skillet, melt the butter over medium heat. Add onions and cook until soft, about 4 minutes, then add the mushrooms and peas, cooking for another minute. Turn the heat to low.
4. Mix the soup, milk and tuna in a separate bowl and add to the skillet. Gently stir until blended together.
5. Add the noodles and the skillet mixture into an oven-proof casserole dish. Mix together. Sprinkle with breadcrumbs.
6. Bake 25-30 minutes. Let stand for 10-15 minutes before serving. Makes 4 adult or 8 preschooler servings.

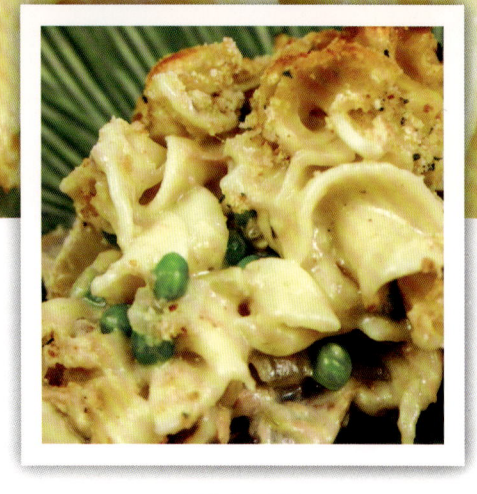

SERVING SIZE

Toddler	¼ cup
Preschooler	½ cup
Adult	1 cup

Nutrition Facts

8 preschooler servings per recipe

Serving size 1/2 cup

Amount Per Serving

Calories 160

	% Daily Value*
Total Fat 6g	8%
Saturated Fat 3g	15%
Trans Fat 0g	
Cholesterol 35mg	12%
Sodium 330mg	14%
Total Carbohydrate 17g	6%
Dietary Fiber 2g	7%
Total Sugars 3g	
Includes 0g Added Sugars	0%
Protein 9g	
Vitamin D 0.6mcg	4%
Calcium 60mg	4%
Iron 1.1mg	6%
Potassium 200mg	4%

* The % Daily Value (DV) tells you how much a nutrient in a serving of food contributes to a daily diet. 2,000 calories a day is used for general nutrition advice.

dinner

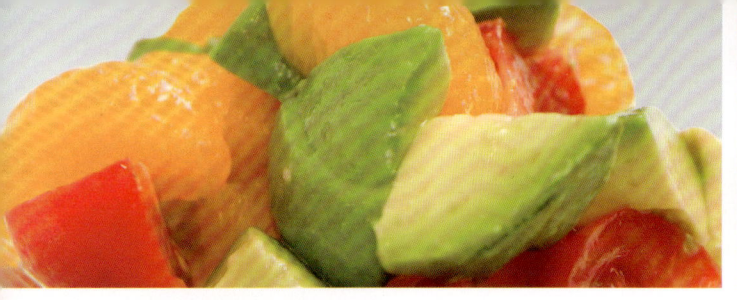

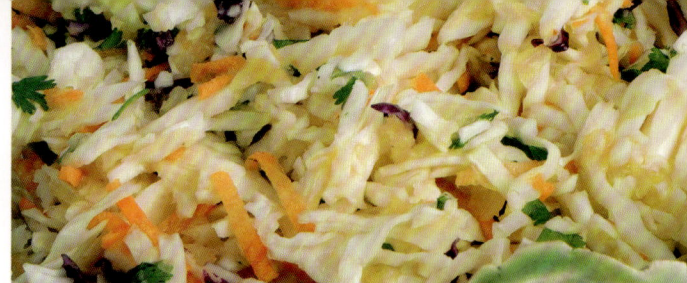

AVOCADO & ORANGE SALAD

HONEY-LIME DRESSING:
2 Tbsp lime juice
1 Tbsp honey
¼ cup olive oil

SALAD:
1 small can (5 oz.) mandarin oranges, drained
1 red bell pepper, diced
1 avocado, diced

DIRECTIONS:
1. In a small bowl, whisk all the dressing ingredients together.
2. In a separate bowl, toss the red pepper and oranges with enough dressing to coat. Add the avocado and gently toss. Serve.

Nutrition Facts Servings: 8, Serv. Size: 1/8
Amount Per Serving: **Calories 130**, Total Fat 11g (14% DV), Sat. Fat 1.5g (8% DV), *Trans* Fat 0g, **Cholest.** 0mg (0% DV), **Sodium** 0mg (0% DV), **Total Carb.** 9g (3% DV), Fiber 3g (11% DV), Total Sugars 7g (Incl. 4g Added Sugars, 8% DV), **Protein** 1g, Vit. D (0% DV), Calcium (0% DV), Iron (2% DV), Potas. (4% DV).

CABBAGE PATCH SLAW

INGREDIENTS:
1 bag (14 oz.) coleslaw mix
¼ cup cilantro, chopped
1 can (8 oz.) crushed pineapple
2 Tbsp lime juice
2 Tbsp honey

DIRECTIONS:
In a medium-sized bowl, toss all ingredients together. Serve.

FISH TACOS!
Make Cabbage Patch Slaw and Pirate Planks (page 49). Serve with tortillas.

Nutrition Facts Servings: 8, Serv. Size: 1/8
Amount Per Recipe : **Calories 35**, Total Fat 0g (0% DV), Sat. Fat 0g (0% DV), *Trans* Fat 0g, **Cholest.** 0mg (0% DV), **Sodium** 0mg (0% DV), **Total Carb.** 9g (3% DV), Fiber 0g (0% DV), Total Sugars 8g (Incl. 4g Added Sugars, 8% DV), **Protein** 0g, Vit. D (0% DV), Calcium (0% DV), Iron (0% DV), Potas. (0% DV).

salads and sides

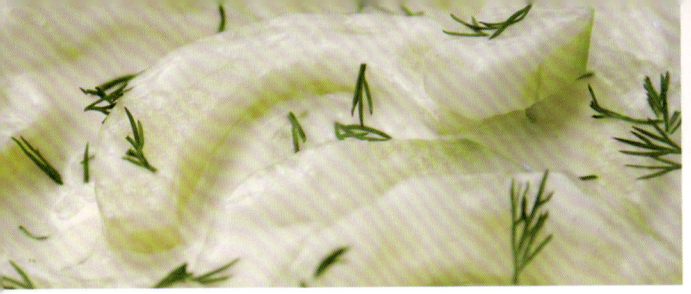

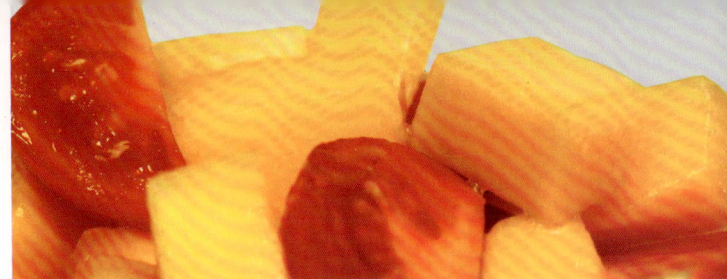

CREAMY "CUKE" SALAD

INGREDIENTS:

2 medium cucumbers, peeled
½ cup plain yogurt
2 tsp apple cider vinegar
2 tsp sugar
1 tsp fresh dill, chopped or ¼ tsp dried dill
Salt and pepper to taste

DIRECTIONS:

1. Cut the cucumbers in half lengthwise. With a small spoon, scrape out the seeds. Slice in ¼-inch thick slices.
2. In a medium-sized bowl, combine yogurt, vinegar, sugar, and dill. Mix together with a spoon until smooth.
3. Add the cucumbers and toss gently to coat the pieces with dressing.
4. Chill until ready to serve.

Nutrition Facts Servings: 8, Serv. Size: 1/8
Amount Per Recipe : **Calories 20**, **Total Fat** 0.5g (1% DV), Sat. Fat 0g (0% DV), *Trans* Fat 0g, **Cholest.** 0mg (0% DV), **Sodium** 10mg (0% DV), **Total Carb.** 3g (1% DV), Fiber 0g (0% DV), Total Sugars 2g (Incl. 1g Added Sugars, 2% DV), **Protein** 1g, Vit. D (0% DV), Calcium (2% DV), Iron (0% DV), Potas. (2% DV).

SWEET TOMATO SALAD

INGREDIENTS:

1 cup fresh tomatoes, cut into bite-sized pieces
1 cup cantaloupe, cut into bite-sized pieces

DRESSING:

¼ cup olive oil or vegetable oil
1 Tbsp lemon juice
1 Tbsp brown sugar
Dash of salt

DIRECTIONS:

1. Place the tomatoes and cantaloupe in a bowl.
2. In a separate bowl whisk together the dressing ingredients.
3. Pour the dressing over the tomatoes and canteloupe and toss to coat.
4. Chill until ready to serve.

Nutrition Facts Servings: 8, Serv. Size: 1/8
Amount Per Serving: **Calories 80**, **Total Fat** 7g (9% DV), Sat. Fat 1g (5% DV), *Trans* Fat 0g, **Cholest.** 0mg (0% DV), **Sodium** 25mg (1% DV), **Total Carb.** 4g (1% DV), Fiber 0g (0% DV), Total Sugars 4g (Incl. 2g Added Sugars, 4% DV), **Protein** 0g, Vit. D (0% DV), Calcium (0% DV), Iron (0% DV), Potas. (2% DV).

salads and sides

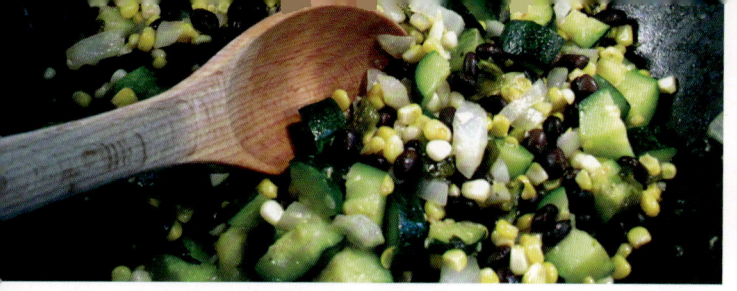

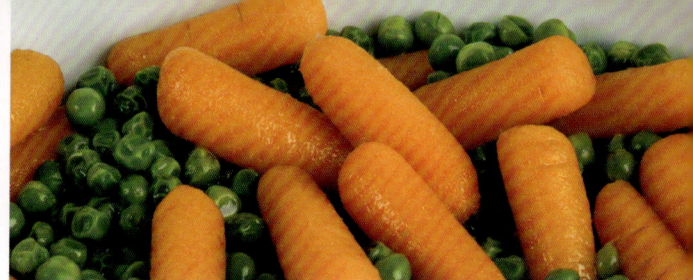

CALABECITAS

INGREDIENTS:

1 can (15 oz.) black beans
2 medium-sized zucchini, diced
½ large onion, diced
1 ½ cups frozen corn
2 Tbsp vegetable oil

DIRECTIONS:

1. Pour the black beans into a colander and rinse for 1 minute under cold water. In a large sauté pan, heat the oil over medium heat.
2. Add the zucchini, onion and corn. Cover stirring occasionally, and cook the zucchini and onion until softened, about 10 minutes.
3. Reduce the heat to low and gently stir in the black beans. Continue cooking until the black beans are heated, about 2 minutes. Serve warm.

Nutrition Facts Servings: 8, Serv. Size: 1/8
Amount Per Recipe : **Calories 140, Total Fat** 6g (8% DV), Sat. Fat 3g (15% DV), *Trans* Fat 0g, **Cholest.** 0mg (0% DV), **Sodium** 210mg (9% DV), **Total Carb.** 17g (6% DV), Fiber 5g (18% DV), Total Sugars 2g (Incl. 0g Added Sugars, 0% DV), **Protein** 5g, Vit. D (0% DV), Calcium (2% DV), Iron (8% DV), Potas. (8% DV).

CANDIED PEAS & CARROTS

INGREDIENTS:

½ pound (about 16) baby carrots
1 cup frozen peas
½ cup water
2 Tbsp butter
2 Tbsp maple syrup

DIRECTIONS:

1. In a saucepan add the baby carrots, peas and water and bring to a boil.
2. Reduce the heat to medium, cover and simmer for 7 minutes. Drain the carrots and peas in a colander.
3. On low heat, add the butter and maple syrup to the saucepan and stir until the butter is melted. Add the peas and carrots and toss gently. Serve.

Nutrition Facts Servings: 8, Serv. Size: 1/8
Amount Per Serving: **Calories 60, Total Fat** 3g (4% DV), Sat. Fat 2g (10% DV), *Trans* Fat 0g, **Cholest.** 10mg (3% DV), **Sodium** 65mg (3% DV), **Total Carb.** 8g (3% DV), Fiber 2g (7% DV), Total Sugars 5g (Incl. 3g Added Sugars, 6% DV), **Protein** 1g, Vit. D (0% DV), Calcium (2% DV), Iron (2% DV), Potas. (2% DV).

salads and sides

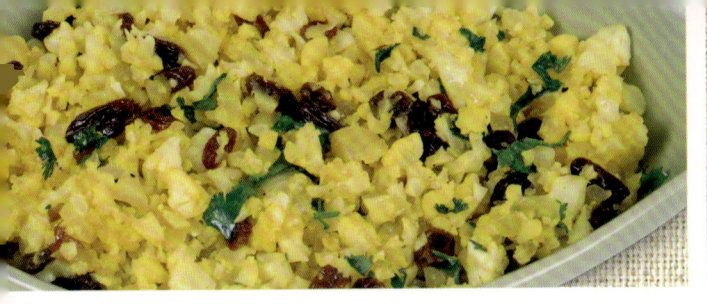

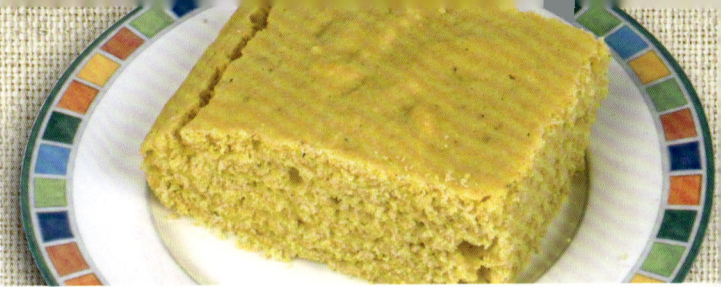

CAULIFLOWER RICE

INGREDIENTS:

1 medium head cauliflower
2 Tbsp vegetable oil
½ medium onion, diced
½ tsp curry powder
¼ cup raisins
¼ cup water
2 Tbsp cilantro, chopped

DIRECTIONS:

1. To "rice" cauliflower: Remove the florets from the stem. Mince florets into tiny pieces.
2. Heat oil and onions in a large skillet over medium heat. Cook and stir the onion until softened, about 4 minutes.
3. Add curry powder, raisins, water and cauliflower. Increase heat to medium-high. Cook about 5 minutes, stirring frequently, until cauliflower is soft, but not mushy. Remove from heat and stir in cilantro. Serve.

Nutrition Facts Servings: 8, Serv. Size: 1/8
Amount Per Serving: **Calories 70, Total Fat** 3.5g (4% DV), Sat. Fat 3g (15% DV), *Trans* Fat 0g, **Cholest.** 0mg (0% DV), **Sodium** 25mg (1% DV), **Total Carb.** 8g (3% DV), Fiber 2g (7% DV), Total Sugars 5g (Incl. 0g Added Sugars, 0% DV), **Protein** 2g, Vit. D (0% DV), Calcium (2% DV), Iron (2% DV), Potas. (6% DV).

CORNBREAD

INGREDIENTS:

1 ¼ cups all purpose flour
¾ cup cornmeal
¼ cup sugar
2 tsp baking powder
1 cup low-fat milk
¼ cup vegetable oil
1 egg
Non-stick cooking spray

DIRECTIONS:

1. Preheat oven to 400°F. Spray 8-inch square baking pan with cooking spray.
2. In a medium-sized bowl, combine the flour, cornmeal, sugar and baking powder. Stir in the milk, oil and egg, mixing until the dry ingredients are moistened.
3. Pour the batter into the baking pan. Bake 20-25 minutes or until light golden brown and toothpick inserted in the center comes out clean.

Nutrition Facts Servings: 9, Serv. Size: 1/9
Amount Per Recipe : **Calories 200, Total Fat** 8g (10% DV), Sat. Fat 6g (30% DV), *Trans* Fat 0g, **Cholest.** 20mg (7% DV), **Sodium** 135mg (6% DV), **Total Carb.** 28g (10% DV), Fiber 1g (4% DV), Total Sugars 7g (Incl. 6g Added Sugars, 12% DV), **Protein** 4g, Vit. D (2% DV), Calcium (8% DV), Iron (8% DV), Potas. (2% DV).

salads and sides

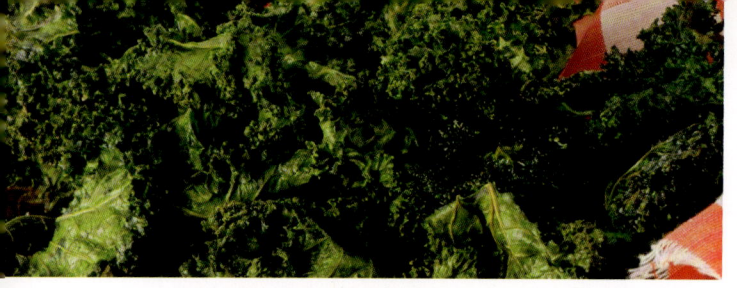

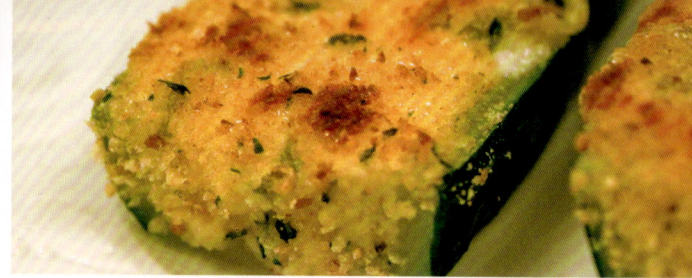

CRISPY KALE

INGREDIENTS:

1 head kale
2 Tbsp vegetable oil
¼ tsp salt

DIRECTIONS:

1. Preheat oven to 300°F.
2. Rinse and dry kale. Remove the center ribs and stems from each leaf. Tear the leaves into 3 to 4-inch pieces.
3. In a large bowl, use your hands to rub each piece of kale with olive oil.
4. Spread kale in single layer on 2 baking sheets lined with foil. Lightly sprinkle with salt.
5. Bake for 18-20 minutes. Remove from oven. Store in an air-tight container for up to 7 days.

Nutrition Facts Servings: 8, **Serv. Size: 1/8**
Amount Per Recipe : **Calories 40**, **Total Fat** 3.5g (4% DV), Sat. Fat 3g (15% DV), *Trans* Fat 0g, **Cholest.** 0mg (0% DV), **Sodium** 80mg (3% DV), **Total Carb.** 2g (1% DV), Fiber <1g (3% DV), Total Sugars <1g (Incl. 0g Added Sugars, 0% DV), **Protein** 1g, Vit. D (0% DV), Calcium (2% DV), Iron (2% DV), Potas. (2% DV).

FROSTED ZUCCHINI

INGREDIENTS:

2 medium zucchini
¼ cup mayonnaise
2 Tbsp green onions, finely chopped
1 tsp lemon juice
2 Tbsp Parmesan cheese
⅛ tsp garlic powder
¼ cup breadcrumbs

DIRECTIONS:

1. Preheat oven to Broil.
2. Cut zucchini in half lengthwise. Steam about 3-4 minutes in microwave until barely tender. Dry on a paper towel and let cool.
3. In a small bowl, mix together remaining ingredients, except the breadcrumbs.
4. Frost one side of the zucchini slice with the mayonnaise mixture. Dip the frosted side in breadcrumbs and place on a foil-lined baking sheet. Broil until lightly browned, about 2 minutes. Serve warm.

Nutrition Facts Servings: 8, **Serv. Size: 1/8**
Amount Per Recipe : **Calories 60**, **Total Fat** 6g (8% DV), Sat. Fat 1g (5% DV), *Trans* Fat 0g, **Cholest.** <5mg (1% DV), **Sodium** 80mg (3% DV), **Total Carb.** <1g (0% DV), Fiber 0g (0% DV), Total Sugars 0g (Incl. 0g Added Sugars, 0% DV), **Protein** 1g, Vit. D (0% DV), Calcium (0% DV), Iron (0% DV), Potas. (0% DV).

salads and sides

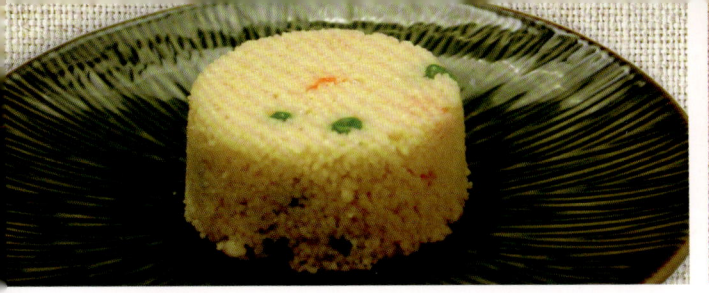

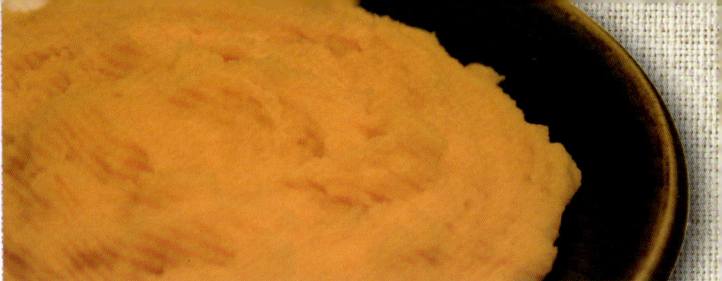

SAND CASTLE COUSCOUS

INGREDIENTS:

1 box (5-6 oz.) couscous
2 Tbsp butter or margarine
½ cup frozen peas and carrots combo
1 small glass bowl or cup
  (this is the mold for your castle)

DIRECTIONS:

Cook both the couscous and peas and carrots separately, according to their package directions. Fluff the couscous with a fork, add the butter or margarine and the vegetables to the couscous and mix gently.

TO MAKE THE SAND CASTLES:

Spoon the mixture into the small bowl or cup. Pack the mixture down using a spoon. Place a plate over the top of the bowl or cup and turn the plate over. Gently remove the bowl or cup. Viola, a sand castle!

Nutrition Facts Servings: 6, Serv. Size: 1/6
Amount Per Recipe : **Calories 160**, **Total Fat** 4.5g (6% DV), Sat. Fat 2.5g (13% DV), *Trans* Fat 0g, **Cholest.** 10mg (3% DV), **Sodium** 60mg (3% DV), **Total Carb.** 24g (9% DV), Fiber 2g (7% DV), Total Sugars 1g (Incl. 0g Added Sugars, 0% DV), **Protein** 5g, Vit. D (0% DV), Calcium (2% DV), Iron (4% DV), Potas. (2% DV).

SMASHED POTATOES

INGREDIENTS:

3 medium-sized white potatoes, peeled
1 medium-sized sweet potato, peeled
5 garlic cloves, peeled
1 can (14 oz.) low-sodium chicken broth
4 Tbsp butter or margarine

DIRECTIONS:

1. Cut potatoes into 2-inch chunks.
2. Place the potatoes and garlic cloves in a saucepan with the chicken broth. Add enough water to cover the potatoes and bring the pan to a boil.
3. Cover and reduce heat to low. Simmer for 20 minutes, until fork tender.
4. Drain the potatoes, saving ¾ cup of the water. Mash the potatoes with a potato masher until they are the same color throughout. Stir in the butter or margarine. Add the saved water ¼ cup at a time, until the potatoes are a creamy consistency.

Nutrition Facts Servings: 8, Serv. Size: 1/8
Amount Per Recipe : **Calories 130**, **Total Fat** 6g (8% DV), Sat. Fat 4g (20% DV), *Trans* Fat 0g, **Cholest.** 15mg (5% DV), **Sodium** 80mg (3% DV), **Total Carb.** 17g (6% DV), Fiber 2g (7% DV), Total Sugars 2g (Incl. 0g Added Sugars, 0% DV), **Protein** 3g, Vit. D (0% DV), Calcium (2% DV), Iron (4% DV), Potas. (8% DV).

salads and sides

ROASTED VEGETABLES

STEP BY STEP: ROASTING VEGETABLES

① Wash vegetables (rinsing for 1 minute under cold water). Preheat oven to 425°F.
② Cut vegetables into same-size pieces.
③ Toss vegetables with 1 tablespoon oil and a light sprinkle of salt and pepper.
④ Spread vegetables onto a pan in a single layer. Put pan in the oven and refer to table below for roasting time.

Vegetables are done roasting when they are fork tender with brown crispy edges.

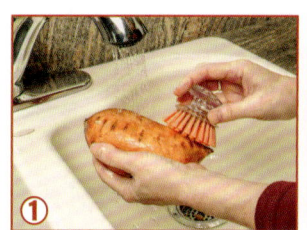

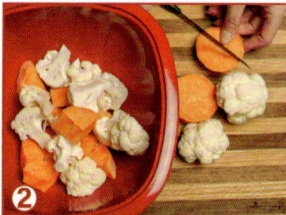

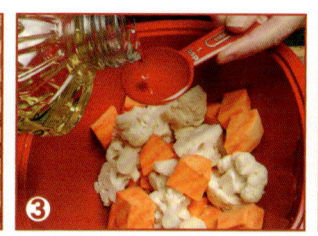

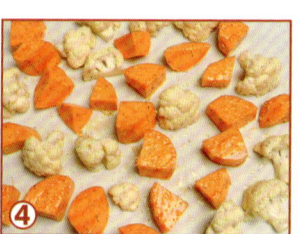

ROASTING TIME	VEGETABLE
15 – 20 minutes	asparagus, bell peppers, green beans, summer squash, tomatoes, zucchini
25 – 30 minutes	broccoli, brussels sprouts, eggplant, mushrooms
40 – 45 minutes	acorn squash, butternut squash, beets, carrots, cauliflower, onions, parsnips, potatoes, yams

salads and sides

STEAMED VEGETABLES

STEP-BY-STEP: STEAMING VEGETABLES ON A STOVETOP

1. Cut vegetables into same-sized pieces.
2. Wash vegetables (rinsing for 1 minute under cold water).
3. Add 1-inch of water to a pot. Set a steamer basket in the pot and add vegetables.
4. Bring to a boil. Cover and reduce heat to medium. Cook 3-5 minutes.

Vegetables are done steaming when they have a bright color and a little crunch.

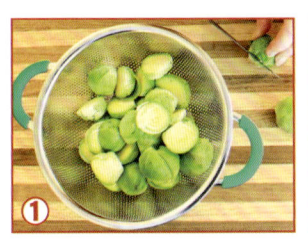

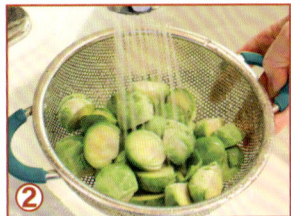

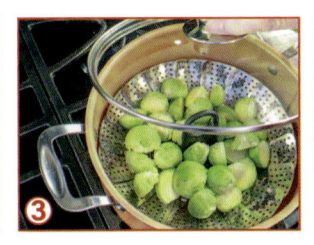

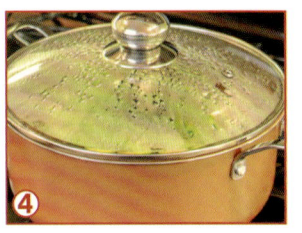

MICROWAVE STEAMING FOLLOW STEPS 1 AND 2 ABOVE THEN...

3. Place vegetables in a microwave-safe dish, cover with plastic wrap and poke 2-3 holes in plastic with a knife.
4. Microwave vegetables on HIGH. Most vegetables will cook in 3-4 minutes.

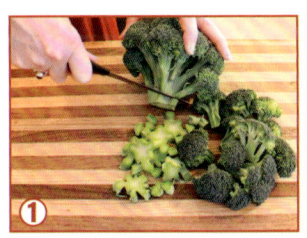

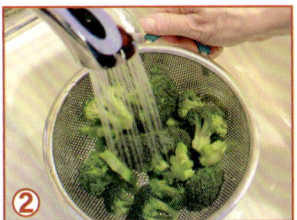

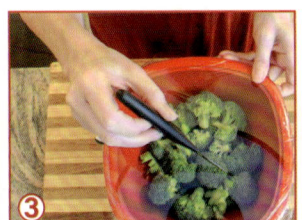

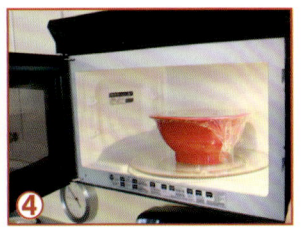

salads and sides

BLACK BEAN SOUP

INGREDIENTS:

1 Tbsp vegetable oil
1 cup onion, chopped
3 garlic cloves, minced
1 can (4 oz.) chopped green chilies
2 tsp ground cumin
2 cans (14 oz. each) diced tomatoes
2 cans (15 oz. each) black beans, drained and rinsed
1 can (15 oz.) low-sodium chicken broth

DIRECTIONS:

1. In a medium-sized pot, heat the oil over medium heat. Add the onion, garlic, cumin and green chilies and cook for 5 minutes.
2. In a blender, combine the onion mixture, tomatoes and beans. Process until smooth.
3. Pour the mixture back into the pot and add the broth. Cook over low heat for about 15 minutes, stirring occasionally. Makes 9 cups.

SOUP BAR:

Serve hot soup with toppings. Each person can choose their favorites. Here are some suggestions:

Sliced green onions	Shredded cheese
Chopped cilantro	Hot sauce or salsa
Avocado cubes	Tortilla chips
Sour cream	Frozen or canned corn

SERVING SIZE

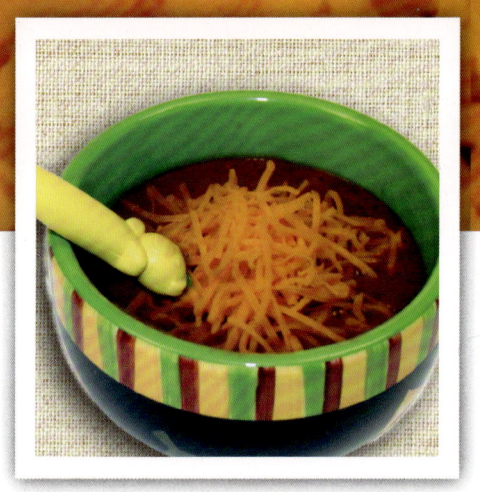

Toddler	½ cup
Preschooler	¾ cup
Adult	1 ½ cups

Nutrition Facts

12 preschooler servings per recipe

Serving size 3/4 cup

Amount Per Serving
Calories 110

	% Daily Value*
Total Fat 1.5g	2%
Saturated Fat 1g	5%
Trans Fat 0g	
Cholesterol 0mg	0%
Sodium 430mg	19%
Total Carbohydrate 18g	7%
Dietary Fiber 6g	21%
Total Sugars 2g	
Includes 0g Added Sugars	0%
Protein 6g	
Vitamin D 0mcg	0%
Calcium 60mg	4%
Iron 2.2mg	10%
Potassium 400mg	8%

* The % Daily Value (DV) tells you how much a nutrient in a serving of food contributes to a daily diet. 2,000 calories a day is used for general nutrition advice.

CREAM OF ASPARAGUS SOUP

INGREDIENTS:

- 2 Tbsp vegetable oil
- ½ cup onion, chopped
- 1 garlic clove, minced
- 1 lb. asparagus, cleaned and chopped
- 1 medium potato, peeled and cubed
- 1 can (15 oz.) low-sodium chicken broth
- 1 cup 2% low-fat milk

DIRECTIONS:

1. In a large soup pot, add oil, onion, and garlic over medium heat. Saute until soft, about 5 minutes.
2. Add asparagus, potato, and broth. Bring to a boil over high heat.
3. Reduce heat, cover, and simmer 20 minutes.
4. Pour in batches into a blender, being careful not to overfill the blender.
5. Puree until smooth. Pour back in the soup pot.
6. Stir in milk. Warm over low heat. Do not boil. Serve. Makes 6 cups.

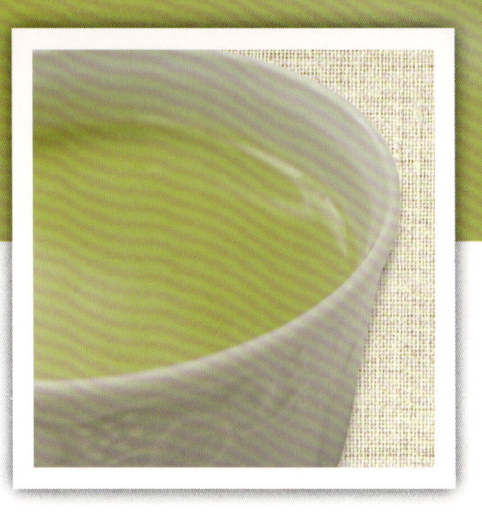

SERVING SIZE

Toddler	½ cup
Preschooler	¾ cup
Adult	1 ½ cups

Nutrition Facts

8 preschooler servings per recipe

Serving size 3/4 cup

Amount Per Serving

Calories 90

	% Daily Value*
Total Fat 5g	6%
Saturated Fat 3.5g	18%
Trans Fat 0g	
Cholesterol <5mg	1%
Sodium 50mg	2%
Total Carbohydrate 9g	3%
Dietary Fiber 2g	7%
Total Sugars 3g	
Includes 0g Added Sugars	0%
Protein 4g	
Vitamin D 0.3mcg	2%
Calcium 60mg	4%
Iron 0.8mg	4%
Potassium 350mg	8%

* The % Daily Value (DV) tells you how much a nutrient in a serving of food contributes to a daily diet. 2,000 calories a day is used for general nutrition advice.

CREAMY CAULIFLOWER SOUP

INGREDIENTS:

1 head of cauliflower, cored and chopped into florets
1 medium potato, peeled and diced
2 cans (15 oz.) low-sodium chicken broth
½ tsp Italian seasoning
2 garlic cloves
1 cup 2% low-fat milk

DIRECTIONS:

1. Place all ingredients in a large soup pot, except the milk.
2. Bring to a boil over high heat.
3. Reduce heat to low, cover, and simmer for 20 minutes.
4. Pour in batches into a blender, being careful not to overfill the blender.
5. Puree until smooth. Pour back in the soup pot.
6. Stir in milk. Warm over low heat. Do not boil. Serve. Makes 6 cups.

SERVING SIZE

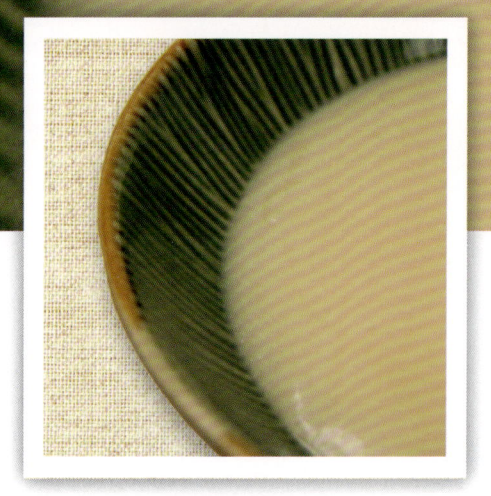

Toddler	½ cup
Preschooler	¾ cup
Adult	1 ½ cups

Nutrition Facts

8 preschooler servings per recipe

Serving size 3/4 cup

Amount Per Serving

Calories 70

	% Daily Value*
Total Fat 1.5g	2%
Saturated Fat 0.5g	3%
Trans Fat 0g	
Cholesterol <5mg	1%
Sodium 80mg	3%
Total Carbohydrate 11g	4%
Dietary Fiber 2g	7%
Total Sugars 3g	
Includes 0g Added Sugars	0%
Protein 6g	
Vitamin D 0.3mcg	2%
Calcium 70mg	6%
Iron 0.7mg	4%
Potassium 490mg	10%

*The % Daily Value (DV) tells you how much a nutrient in a serving of food contributes to a daily diet. 2,000 calories a day is used for general nutrition advice.

LENTIL STEW

INGREDIENTS:

- 1 Tbsp vegetable oil
- 8 oz. Italian sausage
- 1 green pepper, diced
- 1 onion, diced
- 1 medium sweet potato, peeled and diced
- 2 garlic cloves, minced
- 1 cup dry lentils
- 2 cans (15 oz.) low-sodium chicken broth
- 1 (15 oz.) can diced tomatoes

DIRECTIONS:

1. Rinse and drain the dry lentils.
2. In a large pot, heat oil heat over medium-high heat. Add the sausage, and break it up with a wooden spoon while cooking. Cook until browned and no longer pink, 4–6 minutes. Add green pepper, onion, sweet potato and garlic cook about 4 minutes.
3. Add the lentils, chicken broth and tomatoes, bring to a boil.
4. Turn heat to low and simmer for 45-50 minutes until lentils and vegetables are tender, stirring occasionally. Serve. Makes 7 cups.

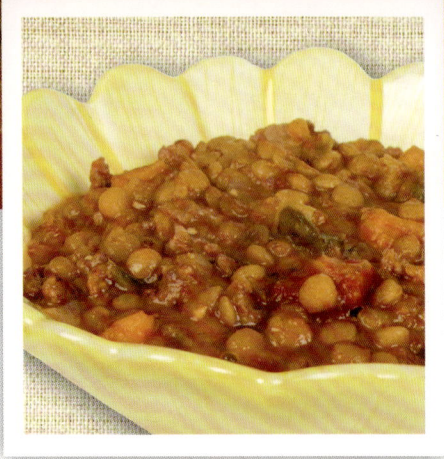

SERVING SIZE

Toddler	½ cup
Preschooler	¾ cup
Adult	1 ½ cup

Nutrition Facts

10 preschooler servings per recipe

Serving size 3/4 cup

Amount Per Serving

Calories 200

	% Daily Value*
Total Fat 9g	12%
Saturated Fat 4g	20%
Trans Fat 0g	
Cholesterol 15mg	5%
Sodium 330mg	14%
Total Carbohydrate 19g	7%
Dietary Fiber 3g	11%
Total Sugars 3g	
Includes 0g Added Sugars	0%
Protein 10g	
Vitamin D 0mcg	0%
Calcium 20mg	2%
Iron 1.8mg	10%
Potassium 340mg	8%

* The % Daily Value (DV) tells you how much a nutrient in a serving of food contributes to a daily diet. 2,000 calories a day is used for general nutrition advice.

soups

WEDDING SOUP

INGREDIENTS:

- 2 quarts (64 oz.) low-sodium chicken broth
- 1 carrot, diced
- 1 celery stalk, diced
- ½ cup small dry pasta, such as elbow or ditalini
- 1 lb. ground pork
- ½ tsp salt and pepper
- ¼ cup parmesan cheese
- ¼ cup breadcrumbs
- 1 can (15 oz.) chick peas (also called garbanzo beans)
- 1 cup green beans, cut (fresh or frozen)

DIRECTIONS:

1. In a large pot, bring the chicken stock, carrot, celery, and pasta to a boil.
2. Turn the heat down to medium and simmer for 10 minutes.
3. While the soup simmers, make the meatballs.
4. In a medium-sized bowl combine the ground pork, breadcrumbs, parmesan cheese, salt and pepper.
5. Roll the meat mixture into ½-inch meatballs.
6. Drop the meatballs into the simmering soup and cook for 5 minutes.
7. Drain and rinse chick peas under cold water for 1 minute.
8. Add the chick peas and green beans to the soup. Cook an additional 5 minutes. Serve. Makes 9 cups.

SERVING SIZE

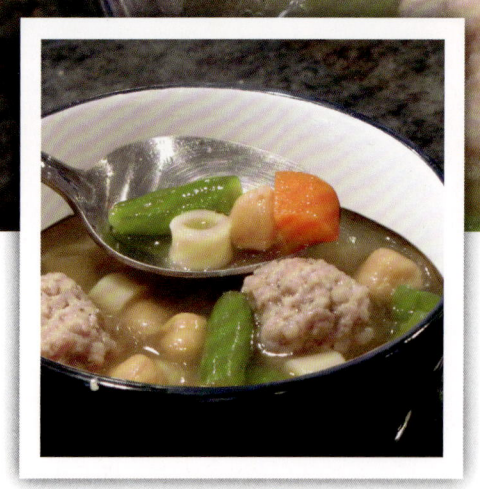

Toddler	½ cup
Preschooler	¾ cup
Adult	1 ½ cups

Nutrition Facts

12 preschooler servings per recipe

Serving size 3/4 cup

Amount Per Serving

Calories 200

	% Daily Value*
Total Fat 9g	12%
Saturated Fat 3.5g	18%
Trans Fat 0g	
Cholesterol 30mg	10%
Sodium 630mg	27%
Total Carbohydrate 15g	5%
Dietary Fiber 2g	7%
Total Sugars 2g	
Includes 0g Added Sugars	0%
Protein 13g	
Vitamin D 0mcg	0%
Calcium 70mg	6%
Iron 1.6mg	8%
Potassium 300mg	6%

* The % Daily Value (DV) tells you how much a nutrient in a serving of food contributes to a daily diet. 2,000 calories a day is used for general nutrition advice.